Chronic Pain
Self-treatment

Including Carpal Tunnel Syndrome

The Schatz Technique™
Brand Pain Prevention *and* Treatment Method

Bernard Schatz, P.T.

Ascara Publishing Company

Edited by Ann Longenecker
All drawings in this book are by the author
Cover design and Graphic and technological support by Daniel Roell
Photos of author and JoAnn Christy by Jim Carpenter
A note from Patch Adams, M.D.
Foreword by Martin P. Albert, M.D.

If you are unable to order this book from your local bookseller, visit the website
www.ReverseYourPain.com

Ascara Publishing Company
#105
536 Pantops Center
Charlottesville, VA 22911

Library of Congress Control Number: 2006908498

ISBN
0-9774707-2-5

Printed in the USA

Have you been told you have Chronic Pain?

2 Questions

1. What **is** Chronic Pain?
2. How Many People Suffer Chronic Pain?

(Answers on next page)

Doctors say if a pain lasts 6 months, it has become "chronic." In other words, the pain is incurable, hopeless. The person will suffer pain the rest of his or her life.

Doctors use the word "chronic" instead of "incurable" or "hopeless" because, well, it *sounds better!* "My doctor just told me I have chronic pain," sounds better than "My doctor just told me that my pain is incurable," or "My pain is hopeless." It helps doctors hide the fact that they are lacking in knowledge. Keep this in mind if your doctor says you have chronic pain.

The gloomy prognosis that dooms millions of people to lives of pain really does spring from a lack of knowledge. I am a physical therapist and have studied and treated chronic pain for over half a century–since I started work in 1950 at the Institute for Medical Research, Cedars of Lebanon Hospital in Los Angeles.

I discovered that the primary cause of chronic pain is contracted tissues that press on nerves. If contracted tissues occur in the neck and scalp, doctors *call* the resulting pain "migraine." If contracted tissues occur in the hand and arm, doctors *call* the pain "carpal tunnel syndrome." And, if contracted tissues occur throughout the body, doctors *call* it "fibromyalgia." **It's all contracted tissues that press on nerves.**

Doctors do not know about contracted tissues–the cause of chronic pain–because they don't examine the *tissues* of people in pain. Instead they carefully study x-rays *of bones.* They may press or prod here or there–but that's not really examining tissues. That's why doctors are lacking in knowledge–why they are unable to reverse the condition that *causes* pain.

I developed a method that *does* reverse the condition that causes chronic pain. The method is described in great detail in this book. It enables people in pain to help themselves to once again have healthy bodies free of pain. **Why "self-treatment for chronic pain?"** *People have to help themselves!* **They can't count on doctors who have already declared their condition to be hopeless.**

How many people suffer chronic pain? According to the American Chronic Pain Association (ACPA) 1 in 3 Americans suffer chronic pain. What a terrible testament to the inadequacy of the medical establishment.

This book is dedicated to the millions
who suffer Chronic Pain needlessly.

IT IS IMPORTANT!

It is important that you have your pain checked out by a doctor before you treat yourself. As discussed throughout this book, doctors do not know how to examine patients for *soft tissue dysfunction* that may be causing chronic pain. They are trained, however, to detect other things, such as vertebral and other fractures, cancer and various disease processes. **The contents of this book are not directed toward these problems and should not be used when they are present.**

By the way, doctors can detect (accurately diagnose) only 20% of what underlies "chronic pain." **The cause of the remaining 80% will remain a mystery to them until they carefully examine the *tissues* of patients in pain.**

Table of Contents

The Schatz Technique™

A Note From Patch Adams, M.D.

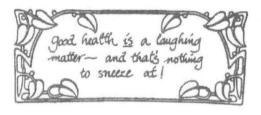

good health is a laughing matter— and that's nothing to sneeze at!

6-23-07

To whom it may concern.

It has been a thrill to get to know Bernard Schatz this year. Reading his book and meeting him I quickly referred a patient to him crippled by chronic pain. He made a long house call and they reported remarkable changes. Bernard has developed his own system to address pain that I wish our hospital were open so that we could fully test it. His compassion is palpable. Give him your attention. In peace

Patch Adams MD

GESUNDHEIT INSTITUTE
6855 Washington Blvd., Arlington, VA 22213
Phone : (703) 525-8169, Fax : (703) 532-6132

A Note From Patch Adams, M.D.

6-23-07

To whom it may concern,

It has been a thrill to get to know Bernard Schatz this year. Reading his book and meeting him I quickly referred a patient to him crippled by chronic pain. He made a long house call and they reported remarkable changes. Bernard has developed his own system to address pain that I wish our hospital were open so that we could fully test it. His compassion is palpable. Give him your attention.

In Peace

Patch Adams M.D.

Foreword

By Martin P. Albert, M.D.

Bernard Schatz has been blessed with many gifts. He is a healer, an artist, an innovator, an original thinker, and a person willing to speak his truth and challenge prevailing practices and beliefs.

I have had the privilege to know Bernard in many capacities–primarily as colleague, but also as physician, client, landlord and ultimately friend. As a colleague I have referred and continue to refer patients to Bernard, and JoAnn Christy, who studied with Bernard and practices "the Schatz Technique." The patients whom I refer are often people with severe, longstanding and unremitting pain, sometimes in a "last resort" situation.

The results of Bernard's treatment are consistently extraordinary. The case histories Bernard describes in this book are consistent with the experiences that my patients have related to me. I have no doubt that the case histories are genuine and accurate. If a patient has the desire to seek treatment with Bernard and to complete a course of therapy, the results are generally gratifying.

Bernard is dedicated to his patients, often charging poor patients minimally for hours and days of treatment. At times Bernard has moonlighted with conventional physical therapy to make ends meet, or has been pulled to other creative outlets to produce the remarkable art that is another of his gifts. But he always comes back to this very unique and effective treatment that he has developed in the course of his career.

Physicians are trained to deal with acute illness. Broken bones, infections, tumors, etc are our forte. Chronic illnesses such as those that produce chronic pain syndromes are not as well handled in a model that is best suited for acute problems. Chronic disease has replaced acute illness as the principle type of health problem that physicians treat, and as the principal cause of disability and reason for use of health care services; chronic illness comprises 78% of health expenses.

The causes of chronic disease are multi-factorial—structural, inflammatory, hormonal, stress related, nutritional, digestion and detoxification related. Addressing chronic disease must necessarily provide interventions for these diverse factors if we are to be successful. These interventions require a team of people with a variety of healing skills, and often manual therapies play a key role in treatment. They take time and patience; they can not be accomplished in a 10 minute visit. They involve participation by the patient in a cooperative effort with the practitioner, and often require actions and changes on the part of the patient.

Bernard has made his life's work understanding and treating the structural changes that occur in soft tissue. These are caused by and, in a viscous cycle, in turn cause further spasm and stiffness, dysfunction and pain. Bernard has mastered the art of finding and gently and persistently treating these "fibrotic" soft tissue changes, thus breaking the cycle of pain and dysfunction in his patients.

We in the medical profession, physicians and others in the healing arts, have much to learn about this dimension of injury and dysfunction that occurs in chronic pain and the incredible possibilities of healing that Bernard's approach offers. The soft tissue changes that Bernard identifies and treats generally are not recognized by physicians trained to look for fractures, tumors, torn ligaments, and positive rheumatoid factors. Thus soft tissue abnormalities associated with pain and inflammation get under the radar of routine medical examination and diagnostic testing, and remain outside the realm of conventional medical attention. As physicians we find what we look for, see what we believe, and like Galileo's inquisitors refuse to look for what we don't believe exists.

As with many aspects of functional medicine approaches to persistent and chronic illness, our challenge as physicians is to bring this work into the arena of what physicians recognize, understand and treat. In this instance, what we need is to bring Bernard's innovative and effective techniques into the mainstream of medical research and therapy. The lack of recognition and interest that Bernard has experienced from physicians in Central Virginia reflects on the malaise of modern conventional medicine—a limited perspective, one-dimensional and reductionist (a single disease has a single cause and this is the same for everyone).

Fortunately, modern conventional medicine also has a strong empirical current and an ongoing commitment to evidence-based science. My hope would be to see outcomes research of Bernard's work. This would confirm its efficacy, and allow the larger medical community to recognize its usefulness and understand the major role that it can have in treating many painful disorders. Indeed, from my observations, Bernard has developed a mode of therapy that in many instances has been more effective than usual conventional care for many pain conditions.

My current wish is to see an apprenticeship program developed which would enable widespread learning and use of this technique by a broad range of people, such as physicians, physical therapists, nurses, and family members of people with chronic pain, as well as the patients themselves. It would be a tragic loss to the healing arts to have these techniques limited to a handful of therapists and a limited number of patients.

Bernard's book is generous in presenting effective treatment approaches to a wide variety of musculoskeletal problems, and timely in meeting a need in the medical profession and society to address chronic painful conditions. That Bernard's work has not been received with serious interest by the medical community is a loss to all of us. Hopefully with this publication, the Schatz Technique will receive broader attention, stimulate outcomes research and clinical trials, provide the recognition due the innovator of an effective healing technique and attract students to learn and disseminate these techniques.

About Martin P. Albert, M.D. and his partner in practice

Dr. Albert's career has included family practice, community medicine, emergency care and teaching medical students at the University of Virginia and the Medical College of Virginia. For the past six years he has intensively studied nutritional, herbal, functional and mind-body approaches to health. He is board certified in Family Practice and in Holistic Medicine, and is certified by the Academy of Guided Imagery. He is on the Visiting Staff of Martha Jefferson Hospital in Charlottesville, VA. Dr. Albert and his wife, Dr. Peggy Wright, created Virginia Integrative Medicine, where they currently practice.

Peggy Wright PhD, RD, CNS has over 20 years experience as a clinician and graduate professor in the field of Complementary and Alternative Therapies. Her education includes bachelor's (UC Berkeley) and master's (Tufts University) degrees in nutrition, and a doctorate in psychology (Saybrook Graduate School) with a specialization in Health, Consciousness, and Spirituality. She recently completed a two-year post-doctoral research fellowship in Complementary and Alternative Therapies at the University of Virginia. Dr. Wright is a Registered Dietitian, a Certified Nutrition Specialist, and a certified Interactive Guided Imagery practitioner.

Drs. Albert's and Wright's skills and experience form a true Integrative Medical Practice. They strive to combine the best evidence-based care from conventional and complementary/alternative medicine. However, they prefer using the more natural and gentler methods of complementary/alternative medicine when possible. Their practice is relationship-centered and emphasizes the patient's active role in healthcare, including lifestyle change and self-care. They recognize the deeper dimensions of healing, including the connection of body, mind, and spirit, and believe that family, community, and the environment play important roles in our overall health and well-being.

Drs. Albert and Wright can be reached at Virginia Integrative Medicine, 901 Preston Avenue, Suites 402-3, Charlottesville, VA 22903. Phone (434) 984-2846. Website: www.healthyvim.org.

(This was written by a patient I treated several years ago. Her name has slipped away from me. If she happens to read this, I hope she contacts me so I can give her credit for it.)

FOR BERNARD SCHATZ, GRATEFULLY

First, take a body that has carried around within it for years cultural and religious messages of: do not feel, do not enjoy. Then add injury and hurt, emotional and physical. The body begins to hunch within itself, cautious, busy as a spider webbing layers of fibers over the wounds.

Walking becomes effortful. Then throw in some adrenaline or heavy lifting. Add a few birthdays. Hurt the back badly once, then over the years, compensate with subtle shifts in carriage, a slight twisting of the torso, an awkward breaststroke kick, to favor the hurt area. Other parts begin to ache. A touch of temporal-mandibular joint pain, persistent stiffness in the shoulders. Forearms ache, too, but this has become steady enough to go unrecognized. The burning in the back becomes a familiar background to motion and work. The head stays busy, thinking, thinking, distracted from the rest.

Then one day, heave a huge potted tree from the ground into the bed of a truck. Astonished by the pain, now slicing hotly down the leg and back up to a point buried deep within the buttock, you walk like a crone. To sit or stand is fearful. Finally, you take your body to meet the shaman.

Gentle, reassuring talk, therapy theory interspersed with joy in the absurd. A reverence for the body, for its mystery. A delight in the creation of healing, at once cocky and humble, funny and awe-inspiring. The humour awakening and soothing at once.

The wise fingers begin their walk.   Hello, here. And hello. And this? Ahhh, right here, I think.

The body's response, instinctive and lasting, is trust.

For two hours, sometimes with talk, sometimes in silence, hands and quiet currents flow over the body, pressing, circling, rotating, finding, finding. The body settles into the shock of feeling itself. Place after place is unerringly identified, pain carried below the level of awareness for so long. Now, gently pointed out with no intense pressure, just shown. This hurts, doesn't it?

The body becomes a map, and for the first time in many years, interesting in its subtleties. Gradual comfort, then an easing of the acute pain, then a yielding of soreness, tightness and unease in shoulder blade, lower back, rib, neck. The mind slows, begins to listen.

Tears threaten. This touching is so simple. Yet the change is so dramatic. The feelings are changing. The feeling of the body is releasing, relaxing, beginning to trust its own structure. The feeling of the heart? The heart is stunned by the gift of this.

Left limply in peace on the table for a few minutes at the end, the room darkened, the healing quietly happens. A rift of decades seals like fractured clay under the potters hands.

The body, the mind, the heart, they are one. They are me.
And I feel BETTER. I flow home.

It all started with Marcia Altscheuler...

I can still remember her name, although it was in 1950 that we met briefly. There is nothing more I recall about her, except she had blonde hair. Strange that I remember her name and the following conversation after all these years.

I had just started classes at Los Angeles City College, and was walking with Marcia. I mentioned to her that I was looking for a job. She said that she had a friend who worked at the Institute for Medical Research, and that one of the labs needed help.

It was this chance remark that set me on the path to search for the cause of chronic pain and how to reverse it.

Or, *was it just a chance remark*? Sometimes I wonder.

The Search For The *Primary* Cause Of Chronic Pain

We are surrounded by a great human tragedy. Millions of people suffer severe, unremitting chronic pain. Their suffering is needless, avoidable and inexcusable.

If you suffer chronic pain, you need to know your suffering does not have to continue and that you can be the one to help yourself to pain-free living. This book will tell you how.

I became a physical therapist a half century ago. In the intervening decades, I have treated hundreds of patients suffering chronic pain, and have worked with doctors, therapists, and other health professionals in numerous work settings.

I have been involved in the study and treatment of chronic pain for over fifty years. Growing up during World War II, I studied photos in *Life* magazine showing the suffering of wounded soldiers and civilians. One photo showed a wounded GI being put into a body cast. The look of agony on his face spoke to me so emotionally that I can still recall it.

In 1950, I became a research assistant at the Cardiovascular/ Renal Dialysis Research Laboratory, Institute for Medical Research, at Cedars of Lebanon Hospital, Los Angeles, California. That same year, I volunteered to stretch the tight limbs of cerebral palsy patients. Thus beginning my half-century study of soft tissue dysfunction. In 1954, I was appointed supervisor of the lab and was distressed by the pain of patients with acute kidney disease and heart problems. This focused my interest in trying to help people who were suffering pain.

In 1957 I graduated from Loma Linda University's School of Physical Therapy. I have experience in numerous areas of physical therapy and rehabilitation: staff physical therapist and supervisor in large rehabilitation centers, hospitals, extended-care facilities, nursing homes, and in-home situations; owner of a large rehabilitation and ancillary-care group; administrator of a home health agency; and a successful practitioner treating chronic pain and physical dysfunction. I have worked with physical therapists, occupational therapists, athletic trainers, orthopedic surgeons, and general practitioners. My passion through the years has been to understand the cause of chronic pain and to develop an effective way to treat it.

At first, I employed the techniques medical mentors taught and continue to promulgate: exercise, stretching, massage, ultrasound, electrostimulation, iontophoresis. However, it soon became clear to me that those modalities had only a temporary, if any, effect in alleviating pain. In fact, some caused an increase in pain. In addition, I noted early on that physical dysfunction was the constant companion of pain. Sufferers reported that their bodies were stiff, weak, and fatigued.

Doctors that dealt with pain were straight-talking in the early days of my training. When a patient with a painful and weak right arm was referred for treatment, the referral bore the simple but honest diagnosis: "painful, weak right arm." Similarly honest diagnoses were given for pain symptoms that occurred elsewhere in the body. Doctors didn't know what caused pain or physical dysfunction and they made no attempt to hide their lack of knowledge. Nowadays, doctors affix impressive-sounding names such as fibromyalgia and repetitive stress disorder onto those same symptoms. These catchy names falsely imply that present-day doctors know more about the cause of pain than their straight-talking predecessors. Dismayed by the severe chronic pain that was minimally affected by the treatments my co-workers and I rendered, and by the equally ineffective drug and surgical treatments doctors administered, I resolved to find more effective ways to treat pain.

I felt there must be a common underlying cause for both the pain and its ever-attendant physical problem, and that, in order for treatment to be effective and long-lasting, it would have to be directed toward that cause, whatever it was. The search for the cause continued for several years.

Then one day I inadvertently applied a more-than-usual amount of lotion to an area I was massaging. When I moved my fingers through the pool of lotion, it was as if a spotlight had been turned on! My fingertips could "see" the tissues inside. In a manner similar to the fingers of the blind discriminating the irregularities of Braille, I now was able to perceive that the painful area I had been working on was composed of tight and contracted skin, fascia, and muscle. By moving my fingers in small circles and varying the pressure, I could distinctly discern each individual tissue system. It was a moment of exciting discovery.

I found that wherever there was a complaint of pain there was also contracted skin, fascia, and muscle. It didn't matter if the pain occurred in the head, neck, forearm, back or leg–it was always accompanied by contracted tissues. Areas that were not contracted were not painful.

With experience, I gained greater expertise, and I learned to use my fingers in a variety of investigative movements that provided additional important information about dysfunctioning tissues. I found that wherever there was a complaint of pain there was also contracted skin, fascia, and muscle. It didn't matter if the pain occurred in the head, neck, forearm, back or leg–it was always accompanied by contracted tissues. Areas that were not contracted were not painful. I also found that the only way the precise character of the underlying tissues could be revealed was by gentle exploration and the use of lotion as a discovering or "connecting" agent. The underlying cause of chronic pain was no longer a mystery.

Now that the precise condition of the tissues that accompanied chronic pain was identified, I developed a technique that would soften and normalize those tissues. Gross massage movements were not delicate enough to be directed toward those specific tissue abnormalities my discovery agent and examining fingers disclosed. A technique that explored and softened each tissue system was required. Over the next several years, I developed and refined this technique. When gently applied, tight tissues softened, became normal, and pain went away! My search for the cause of chronic pain, wherever it occurs in the body, and real treatment of the cause, had ended in success.

I concluded that contracted tissues tightly grip and squeeze pain receptors, nerves, and blood vessels, thereby causing the symptoms of pain, fatigue, and weakness. I learned that to achieve full recovery, all tissue systems have to be examined, treated and normalized. In the following years, I successfully treated the cause of pain throughout the body, including those types of pain with recently acquired impressive names. Patients who had been told they would have to suffer chronic pain for the rest of their lives became pain-free and stayed pain-free because the underlying problem had been normalized. My treatment enabled patients to avoid surgery that had been ordered. Other patients were returned to pain-free health after unsuccessful surgeries had been performed.

In addition to being a medical researcher and physical therapist, I am also an artist, primarily a sculptor. In 1986, 1 won a coveted position as artist-in-residence at the Roswell Museum of Art in Roswell, New Mexico. It is natural for me to use my hands as a sculptor and also as a means of examining and treating patients suffering pain. My background as a researcher and my artistic freedom enabled me to develop a treatment approach from an independent point of view, not one locked into myths, misconceptions, and erroneous notions.

All areas of the body are interrelated and interconnected, making up a continuum. Thinking of the head as being separate and apart from the neck, and the neck as being separate and apart from the shoulder, is arbitrary and misleading. Unfortunately, the medical community has fallen into this fragmented concept of the human body. A problem with the knee or thigh is viewed as being separate and apart from a problem with the low back or gluteal region.

I asked my thirteen-year-old daughter, Anna, if it sounded reasonable to her that "if one part of the body is dysfunctional, then all parts of the body become dysfunctional."

She answered, "Well, if one part of the body is hurt, then the part right next to it gets affected, and then the part right next to that gets affected, then the part right next to that gets affected, and so on, until the whole body gets affected."

This leads me to offer a cautionary note about this book. When I describe problems with different "parts" of the body, it is with the understanding that these "parts" are, in reality, segments of a continuum. I have separated out these continuum segments for convenience of discussion only. It is quite different when I treat, or when other practitioners should treat, patients suffering chronic pain. The next time you discuss soft tissue dysfunction with your doctor, mention Anna's theory. It might expand your doctor's horizons.

Our bodies are marvelously complex, and their workings are difficult to fathom. I make no claim to understand more than just a very tiny bit of how they function. The condition of our tissues is determined by the confluence of a great number of internal and external factors. Physical and emotional "insults" or injuries stimulate tissue dysfunction, but nutritional deficiencies, environmental and societal stressors, mental attitudes, and other factors of which I am unaware must also play a part.

It is important that dysfunctioning tissues are normalized, not only to eliminate pain, but also because contracted tissues squeeze vascular and neurologic structures; they interfere with the flow of normal processes, thus causing the health of the individual to become degraded. As tight, contracted tissues contribute to organ disease, I am confident that eventually everyone will be examined and treated for tissue dysfunction, because the relationship of contracted tissues and the state of one's health will be firmly established in the future.

Naturally, I was excited by my successes and attempted to share what I had learned with doctors and co-workers. To my surprise, the message of real treatment was met with a profound lack of interest. It eventually became evident that doctors did not welcome guidance from someone outside their profession, and fellow therapists chose not to question the authority of physicians.

Sadly, patients today with chronic pain continue to receive what they believe are treatments but in reality are merely methods that attempt to manage, that is, reduce the severity of their complaints. Until doctors understand their unseen enemy, they will joust ineffectively with its painful effects. This will continue until doctors learn how to properly examine patients experiencing chronic pain. Doctors use X-rays to examine the **bones** of patients suffering chronic pain. However the **tissues** of chronic pain sufferers have to be carefully examined to find contracted areas–the cause of their pain.

The medical community's attempt to deal with the *secondary* symptom of pain by the use of drugs, surgery, or other means without treating the underlying cause is doomed to failure, a failure that has become abundantly evident in the current epidemic of pain and suffering. The endless ads on TV touting pain relievers, including "doctor-recommended" ones, are constant reminders that doctors do not understand what is causing pain or how to treat it.

Doctors can find the exact cause, such as a structural abnormality, in only a small percentage of chronic pain. The underlying cause of the vast majority of chronic pain remains a mystery to the medical community. I contend that this mysterious cause is unidentified soft tissue dysfunction.

After years of frustrating attempts to have doctors understand why their patients are suffering and that real treatment is available, I finally gave up on them. Instead, I decided to write a book directed not toward doctors, but toward the pain sufferers themselves. If what I write rings true, they will know they no longer have to suffer pain; they can help themselves.

Because of their ineffective focus on secondary symptoms, doctors have grown pessimistic and say what they call migraine, fibromyalgia, and chronic pain are incurable. Doctors' defeatist attitudes eclipse the truth of great hope for those who suffer chronic pain. The cause of your pain can be treated and your body can be healed. The message of this book is that you do not have to give up; you can heal yourself of your pain.

In this book, you are given important information and detailed drawings that will enable you to locate the tissues that are causing your pain. A treatment technique, developed over a forty-year period, that normalizes the cause of pain is carefully described. Fifty case histories that demonstrate the success of real treatment are presented.

You will learn that tight, contracted tissues result from emotional stress turned inward, as well as from physical insults and trauma. These effects accumulate throughout the body. As they do, some areas become particularly tight, causing pain. If one of these areas happens to be the neck and head, doctors call the resulting pain migraine; if the hand and forearm, carpal tunnel syndrome; and if throughout the body, fibromyalgia.

When you finish reading this book, you will have a thorough understanding of soft tissue dysfunction, which is the primary cause of chronic pain, and will know how you can treat yourself so your body can heal. Your pain will go away and stay away.

PART ONE:

What *Causes* Chronic Pain?

Soft Tissue Dysfunction:

The *Primary* Cause of Chronic Pain

Chronic pain is not beamed into your body from some mysterious cloud overhead. For every complaint of pain there is an area of the body that has tight and contracted tissues. The dysfunctioning tissues press on pain receptors. Release the tight tissues, and pain goes away and stays away.

All cells and tissues of creatures of the animal kingdom share a commonality. They are all programmed to contract as a response to being irritated. From the single-celled amoeba to the cell colony of the jellyfish to the cells that make up the tissues of mankind, cells and tissues contract when irritated. This inherent tendency of the soft tissues of our body to contract is the primary cause of our chronic pain.

When an area of the body is insulted by injury, overuse, or by any physical or emotional stress, the tissues of that area react by going into spasm. Once tissue becomes spasmed, it stays that way–it is unable to release itself. Over time, the injured area becomes tighter and tighter. This process continues for days, weeks, months, or years. As time passes, spasmed tissue loses its healthy suppleness and gradually changes into thick, unhealthy tissue that constricts the blood vessels and nerves passing through it.

The dysfunctioning tissue triggers other areas of the body to become tight and contracted. The individual gradually adjusts or accommodates to what is happening to her body and is unaware how much her body has changed.

The person may have episodes or flare-ups of pain that come and go. But after a visit to her doctor and a prescription for stronger pain reliever, she is assisted to a higher level of dysfunction. Her pain may seem to go away but really does not; she merely adjusts to a new level. More time passes, more thickening happens, more pain receptors get squeezed tighter and tighter. More accommodation happens, more adjusting to having larger areas of the body affected and in pain.

After five, ten, fifteen years or more of this, extensive areas of the body have changed into thickened, scarlike tissue. Because we accommodated to them as they developed, we are unaware of them.

However, those flare-ups of pain do catch our attention, and doctors give them names. But they are, after all, merely symptoms of the underlying cause: tight, contracted tissue. Unless the underlying cause is dealt with, symptom after symptom will continually appear. Fortunately, just as every tissue has the ability to contract, the same tissue also has the potential of having the process reversed, of becoming supple and healthy and pain-free again, but only if appropriate treatment is given.

What Are Soft Tissues?

The term soft tissue can be confusing. Anatomically speaking, the body is divided into two types of tissues: hard tissues (the bones), and soft tissues (everything else).

The problem is that soft tissues can become tight and contracted, i.e., hardened. This means you can have hard "soft" tissues. The soft tissues of the body that are primarily involved with chronic pain are:

1. skin
2. muscles
3. fascia
4. ligaments

These tissues have a strong potential of becoming severely contracted. Tendons, though frequently made out by doctors to be responsible for body pain and physical dysfunction, are rarely a cause for concern. They are tough and lie in protective sheaths that are well lubricated. Their reputation for causing body dysfunction springs from a lack of knowledge of body tissues.

Let's look at what happens to these four tissue systems that become major components of chronic pain and physical dysfunction.

1. **Skin.** Healthy skin is soft and supple. It is easily moved over tissues that lie under it. It does not hurt when gently pressed. When skin is triggered to become dysfunctional, it tightens and thickens. It gets stuck to the tissues that lie under it. Pain is elicited when it is gently touched. The skin of the entire body may become tight and contracted, making all movements painful and difficult.

   Dysfunctioning skin is a major component of hand and finger problems. It presses down on the joints of the fingers and thumb, contributing to stiffness and pain. The skin of the palm thickens and grows taut, causing the entire hand to become stiff and unable to function properly. One sees residents of nursing homes dependent on others because of this.

   Skin overlying the area of the carpal tunnel at the base of the palm, when triggered to become dysfunctional, thickens and develops an almost plastic-like hardness. It becomes stuck to the fascia and ligament that form the roof of the tunnel, thus contributing to the problems there.

   An area of skin dysfunction that can have particularly serious health consequences is that of the lower extremity. Tight, contracted skin overlying the calf is frequently a component of peripheral vascular disease. The calf of someone suffering arterial insufficiency will invariably be found to have skin that is extremely hard, tight, and contracted, having an almost wooden feel. The skin is tightly adherent to the tissues underneath. This produces a tourniquet effect that squeezes arterial vessels, making their job of supplying blood to the tissues of the leg increasingly difficult. The result is not only severe pain, but also tissues that are so unhealthy that ulcers develop. The tissues may become so severely damaged and life-threatening that amputation is eventually required.

If the skin anywhere on the body is thick, tight, adherent to underlying tissues or structures, and is painful to the touch, it is unhealthy and is a strong indicator that the tissues underlying it are also unhealthy. The skin and the unhealthy tissues under it need to be treated so the individual can become healthy and pain free again.

2. **Muscles.** The purpose of skeletal muscle tissue is to shorten in length, thereby causing the joint to which it is connected to move. Healthy muscles are able to relax and lengthen again after this contractive action. When stressed, muscles progressively lose their normal ability to lengthen and *remain* in the contracted stage. They squeeze pain receptors, nerve endings that transmit the sensation of pain, and pain is generated. As time goes on, and they get tighter and more contracted, they become bound down by fibrotic tissue (which will be discussed in a moment).

   As years pass, the individuals feel more pain, grow weaker, and find movement difficult. They are told this is "merely something that happens with old age." This is not true. The truth is that this is what happens when a soft tissue problem is not properly treated. More than that, it is what happens when the present healthcare system is so tragically unaware of soft tissue dysfunction that a problem that could have been easily treated years earlier is allowed to worsen and cause lifelong pain, suffering, and premature debility.

3. **Fascia.** Fascia is a type of tissue that is found throughout the body. It is a thin, strong tissue similar in appearance to Saran Wrap, but much more

pliable. It provides protective boundaries to the softer body tissues. Healthy fascia conforms easily to the ever-changing shapes of soft tissues as the various parts of the body constantly move. When fascia is stimulated to become dysfunctional, it thickens, tightens, and contracts. Instead of protecting the soft tissues it surrounds, it binds them and restricts their movement.

As time passes and fascia grows thicker and more contracted, the soft tissues of the body become increasingly stiff. Movement becomes painful and difficult. Yet with proper treatment this process can be reversed, and thick, tight, contracted fascia can become soft, supple, and healthy again.

4. **Ligaments.** Strong bands called ligaments hold the joints of the body together. When ligaments are in a healthy condition, they allow the joints to move freely. However, when stimulated to become thick and contracted, they tighten down on the joints, restricting their movement and stressing the joint structure. If proper treatment is not provided and the stress is allowed to continue over an extended period, the joint may become so painfully damaged that it has to be replaced with a mechanical one.

All four tissue systems–skin, muscles, fascia, ligaments–must be examined, treated, and normalized if complete recovery is to be achieved.

The Fibrotic Fiber

So far, dysfunctioning tissue has been described as being tight and contracted. But we now have to discuss an additional and very important element of tissue dysfunction.

When the body is injured or stressed, tiny fibers appear throughout the injured area. I do not know how these fibers form or what their composition is, but I know they are there because I can feel them. I call them "fibrotic fibers" because I contend they are associated with a condition called "fibrosis," a thickening of tissues. My awareness of them started several years ago when I began using lotion as a discovering agent and the tiny subunits of the contracted tissue were revealed.

Since then, I have refined my perception of these fibers and realize that they coalesce to form a variety of shapes and sizes. These range from tiny hair-like configurations, to round, hard knots almost like ball bearings, to cable-like forms as thick as a thumb found in the gluteal and upper thigh areas.

When the body is injured or stressed, tiny fibers appear throughout the injured area. I call them "fibrotic fibers" because I contend they are associated with a condition called "fibrosis," a thickening of tissues. When groups of fibrotic fibers fuse, they become the thick formations one finds in advanced cases of tissue dysfunction.

The more advanced the tissue dysfunction, the greater the aggregate of fibrotic fibers. I believe these fibrotic fibers are sent out by the body to strengthen an area that is under physical or emotional stress, much as immune T cells are sent out to defend an area of the body that is under stress of infection.

When groups of fibrotic fibers fuse, they become the thick formations one finds in advanced cases of tissue dysfunction. I am speaking of the hard tissue that binds down the joints of hands and fingers; or the thick tissue of the sternocleidomastoid muscle where it attaches behind the ear; or the plastic-like tissue overlying an unhealthy carpal tunnel.

When treating someone who has areas of thick, contracted fibrotic tissue, I find that as treatment progresses, these areas of dysfunction fragment into their subcomponent forms. Finally, the individual fibers soften and disappear. The area once again is normal, healthy, and free of pain.

What Does Cumulative Trauma Feel Like?

The terms "cumulative trauma" and "repetitive stress injury" are frequently bandied about by doctors. But just what accumulates when tissues are repetitively stressed is not mentioned. I contend it is the progressive

8

accumulation of fibrotic fibers. The greater the accumulation, the thicker the area and the more severe the symptoms.

It is difficult to precisely describe the shape and texture of fibrotic tissue, fibrotic structures, and fibrotic fibers. You have to actually feel them. Terms such as "ropy," "ball bearing-like," or "cable-like" are the best I have come up with. It is equally difficult to describe the sensations that are elicited when these areas and structures are treated and released. Expressions such as "an itchy feeling," "a feeling of release," "it feels lighter," "it feels looser," "it feels better," "a feeling like electricity" are the best my patients have come up with.

When Does Soft Tissue Dysfunction Start?

By the time a person first becomes aware that he is having chronic pain, the development of extensive soft tissue dysfunction is well under way.

Long before the individual goes to a doctor's office and is given pain pills for backache, sinus pain, or migraines, his body has profoundly changed. As years go by and he returns for stronger medication, his body continues to change, to become increasingly tight, contracted, and fibrotic.

It is my contention that this process starts early in childhood and continues throughout the lifetime of the individual. I believe it is the result of repeated physical and emotional insults that stimulate the body to form and accumulate fibrotic tissue. I have had the opportunity to examine and treat children ten years of age or younger and have found well-developed soft tissue dysfunction in these children. Maybe "growing pains" should not be ignored after all!

The development of dysfunctioning tissue begins after any emotional or physical insult to the body. The emotional insult can result from being scolded by a parent or teacher, the stress of driving in traffic, or trouble at work with the boss. Physical insults can be from outright trauma, such as car accidents, stumbling in a playground or falling out of a tree. It can take the form of postural stress, such as happens to students bending forward with heavy packs on their backs, or it can can result from overuse, as happens to dancers, musicians, and computer operators.

An emotional or physical insult directed to any part of the body causes the tissues in that part to spasm. If the spasm is not treated, released, and normalized, it develops into the next stage: contraction. If this stage is not treated, it develops into fibrotic tissue.

Physical and emotional insults can be very subtle and cause only minute spasm reactions. But the results can accumulate throughout a lifetime. Thus, tissue dysfunction started in early childhood and continued throughout adolescence and young adulthood can result in profound pain and disability in later life.

In caveman days, if you were in a stressful situation–say a saber-toothed tiger was attacking you–you either ran away or grabbed a club and fought your way out of the situation. To enable your muscles to have the extra energy needed to fight or run, nature provided you with a fight-or-flight system. This system, part of the autonomic nervous system, gives you the big spurt of energy you need to pull yourself out of emergency situations.

In the old days, those "energy chemicals" were dissipated by the activity of running or fighting. Today when we are in a stressful situation, we are not afforded the opportunity of using up those chemicals. They are turned inward and cause our muscles to tighten. With each little spurt of energy chemicals released with each little stressful situation we are confronted with, our muscles and their associated tissues tighten a bit more. Over a lifetime, the accumulation of all these tightenings contributes to the tissue dysfunction that underlies your chronic pain.

Hidden Pain

You may have lived with pain so long you don't know how much you are hurting! In order to just survive, your body has learned how to accommodate to pain, how to block out much of your pain. We now need to discuss something I call "hidden pain."

Hidden pain occurs when your body is subjected to very slowly increasing amounts of physical or emotional stress. Let us say, for example, that the tissues of your shoulder are insulted in some manner.

As a response, your shoulder tissues tighten just a "teeny-tiny" bit. This teeny-tiny bit of tightening squeezes just a teeny-tiny amount on the pain receptors located within its tissues. These pain receptors relay the teeny-tiny pain message on to your pain-sensing center. (The pain sensing system is marvelously complex. For purposes of illustration, I simply call it the "pain-sensing center.")

The pain-sensing center dismisses the teeny-tiny message of pain from your shoulder. The pain-sensing center has a capability of blocking out trifling amounts of pain signals that come to it from the various parts of your body. This ability to accommodate to small levels of pain allows the pain-sensing center to concentrate on more dramatic items coming to it.

You have now successfully accommodated to that teeny-tiny bit of pain. You are no longer aware of it. You no longer perceive it. But the tissues at your shoulder continue to tighten just a teeny-tiny bit more. The pain receptors are squeezed just a little bit more. Again, your pain-sensing center receives the signal and easily accommodates to it. The small amount of increased pain is again blocked out.

This process of accommodating to, of blocking out messages of very small increments of pain, continues day in, day out, month in and month out, year in and year out. Although you are not consciously aware of it, you have accumulated large amounts of pain that have been stored up in the tissues of your body.

The accommodation process is not perfect. You may be aware of aches and pains here and there that come and go. When pain messages are more intense than usual, you may be aware of severe flare ups of pain. Your body eventually accommodates, more or less successfully, to even these episodes, particularly if your doctor gives you pain medicine to tide you over. This is why you are not aware of how much pain there is in your body.

By the way, you are not aware of something else that has slowly been happening to your body. You have not noticed the imperceptible tightening that caused the accumulation of hidden pain. You are not aware of just how stiff and unhealthy your body has gradually become.

Hidden pain areas are difficult to describe. They need to be experienced. Here is how you may experience them: put some lotion on, say, your left forearm. Any body lotion will do for this experiment. Lotions are discussed in greater detail later in the book. Move the fingers of your right hand in slow, firm, but gentle circles on the lotioned skin of the forearm. Very gently squeeze the skin of your forearm just below your elbow. You will soon find areas of your skin and the tissues underneath your skin that are surprisingly painful (if this is a dysfunctioning area). In fact, you hadn't known they were painful at all.

As you explore your lotioned tissues, you will be further surprised at the variety and extent of your hidden pain areas. Some will elicit a dull, aching sensation; some will be intensely tender and painful. But all will have been hidden from your conscious awareness before you applied the lotion and performed your gentle explorations.

To sum up, hidden pain areas are components of the body's mechanism that allows us to accommodate to progressive soft tissue dysfunction. Or rather, they are a *result* of the body having successfully accommodated itself to prolonged periods of incremental pain and dysfunction.

TCF Relay Points

TCF ("Tight, Contracted, Fibrotic," a term I have coined) relay points are small areas of compressed tissue that relay the perception of pain to points in other areas. When a TCF relay point is pressed, pain is felt at that particular point and is also perceived at one or more distant areas.

It is interesting to note the unique pattern of TCF relay points. Just as snowflakes are different, one from the other, so are the patterns of TCF relay points from one individual to another. For example, if you press on a particular spot on one individual (say an inch below the left elbow), pain may be perceived on the back of the index finger of the left hand. If you press on exactly the same area of another individual, pain may be felt at the shoulder, chest, or some other part of the body. TCF relay points appear to be components of the transmission system that allows one area of soft tissue dysfunction to stimulate other areas to become unhealthy.

The Five Axioms of Soft Tissue Dysfunction

First Axiom: All body tissues have a potential, a capability to contract.

Second Axiom: Soft tissue can be insulted in two ways: by emotional stress, or by physical trauma.

Third Axiom: When soft tissue is insulted a process is started that continues inexorably from spasm, to contraction, and finally fibrosis.

Spasm. In the first stage of the process, an area of the body has been insulted. The tissues of that specific area react by going into spasm. Pain receptors are squeezed, irritated, and send out signals of pain that the body accommodates to. Vascular and neurological supply is still adequate.

Contraction. In the second stage of the process, gradually, over a few to several months, the spasmed tissues have developed into a more tightened state. Pain receptors are increasingly irritated. The body attempts to accommodate to the increased intensity of these pain signals, and hidden pain areas develop. Vascular and neurological structures are squeezed. Other tissue areas are triggered to become spasmed and contracted. These additional areas squeeze and irritate their pain receptors, resulting in yet additional areas of tightness and pain. The problem has become "global."

Fibrosis. More time goes on and the contracted tissue becomes thicker and tougher. It takes on a scar-like consistency; fibrotic development has started. Vascular and neurologic circulation becomes strangled. There is more accommodation to increasing pain, and therefore, increasing accumulation of hidden pain areas. As the years roll on, the body becomes increasingly unhealthy and dysfunctional. Organ systems are affected; joint structures, reacting to the continued stress, become damaged; skin becomes thickened, hardened, and indurated; movement becomes difficult. The individual becomes depressed and quality of life is significantly reduced. The problem has become what the medical community calls "chronic."

Fourth Axiom: Once contracted, body tissue cannot uncontract; it cannot normalize itself.

Fifth Axiom: Just as all tissues are susceptible to a *process* that causes them to become contracted, so too are they susceptible to having this process reversed. With proper treatment, contracted and fibrotic tissue can once again become normal, supple, and healthy. Doctors are mistaken in their belief that when the condition has become "chronic" it is "incurable," and the sufferer must be consigned to the hopeless bin and referred to the hell of pain management centers.

Of course, the earlier effective treatment is initiated, the more likely complete success can be achieved. However, even after tissue dysfunction has been allowed to worsen for year after year, dramatic reversals are still likely, and significant improvement in the most advanced cases is the expected outcome.

How In The World Can Doctors Know Why Their Patients Are Hurting, If they Don't Carefully Examine Their Tissues?

Medical "Treatment" of Chronic Pain:
Dangerous Drugs, Mutilating Surgery, and .... Deadening of Nerves

An Overview

Never assume that doctors who deal with chronic pain possess great knowledge or do things in a "scientific way."

Did you know that doctors consider "chronic pain" to be a *hopeless* condition? If a pain continues for more than a few months, doctors feel it has become permanent. They call this *chronic* (no hope of recovery) *pain*. Keep this in mind if you have been told that *you* have chronic pain. It means that doctors have dumped you into the Hopeless Bin, and have condemned you to suffer pain for the rest of your life.

Doctors don't have the courage and honesty to look a patient in the eye and say they consider the case to be "hopeless." Instead, they tell pain sufferers that they have "chronic pain."

Doctors involved in heart and brain surgery have developed greatly improved techniques and treatments. So have cardiologists, urologists, dermatologists, ophthalmologists, and those that treat cancer. Doctors practicing in most branches of medicine have achieved results worthy of praise.

Doctors dealing with chronic pain are the exception to the rule--their patients *continue* to suffer. Their failure to effectively treat chronic pain springs from their profound lack of knowledge of soft tissue dysfunction.

Doctors dealing with chronic pain are good memorizers. The ability to memorize enabled them to memorize the material their teachers presented in their early schooling, thus getting high grades, which in turn got them into medical school. Being such good memorizers, these doctors memorized all the myths and misconceptions relating to chronic pain that were written in their medical textbooks, instead of thinking things through for themselves and developing better methods of treating their patients.

Don't Throw the Patient out the Window

I had a professor of neurology who would jocularly admonish his students, "Class, study your textbooks! Study, study your textbooks! And when you are out in practice and have a patient that doesn't fit your textbook, throw the *patient* out the window."

Unfortunately, this is just what medical practitioners are doing when someone comes to them with chronic pain. They have been trained to think along certain lines, to examine their patients in certain ways, to prescribe certain drugs, to perform certain surgeries. They have studied their textbooks well and continue to throw their patients out the window.

These doctors **see** only what they have been trained to see, and **hear** only what they have been trained to hear. When they diagnose someone as having carpal tunnel syndrome, they see only the wrist. They do not see all the obvious and dramatic signs of dysfunction that occur throughout the entire upper extremity. They hear only the complaints that pertain to the wrist. They do not hear the complaints of pain that occur outside that very narrow band.

The history of medical practitioners displays ample evidence of arrogant specialist mind-set. For just one example, let us look at what medical experts in Australia and the United States did to victims of polio in the 1930s. They immobilized weakened limbs in rigid and excruciatingly painful plaster casts, and arrogantly disregarded any other treatment approach. These medical specialists attacked and pilloried Sister Kenny, a nurse, when she demonstrated effective and humane treatment. It was not until thousands of victims had been tortured and denied an opportunity for recovery that these so-called experts were forced to change their ways.

So it is with the medical community of today, that segment dealing with chronic pain. These self-proclaimed experts are looking in the wrong direction when their patients complain of pain. They have created a rigid concept, a rigid model. Anything that does not fit into this model is disregarded, with disastrous results for their patients.

Medical "Treatment" of Chronic Pain: Dangerous
Drugs, Mutilating Surgery, and .... Deadening of Nerves.

I have tried many times over the years to get doctors to carefully touch their patients so they would understand why their patients are hurting; however, they have always been so reluctant to do so that I failed in my attempts.

Recently, I attended the neurologic exam of one of my patients. I wanted his neurologist to feel the areas I was working on. I had a tube of lotion with me and applied some to an area of tissue dysfunction.

"Feel how tight, how fibrotic this tissue is, doctor," I said, as I moved my fingers through the lotion. But the doctor declined to touch the lotioned skin of his patient. "Feel *this* area," I repeated, applying lotion to another area of dysfunction. Again, the doctor declined to touch his patient. This time, I took the doctor's hand and gently moved it in circular motions so his fingers could feel the fibrotic tissue. But the doctor immediately withdrew his hand and wiped off the small amount of lotion that had gotten onto his fingers. It was as if it was beneath his dignity to touch the skin of his patient.

I have done this sort of thing, from time to time, with other doctors, trying to get them to feel what I had carefully described in my reports to them about their patients. But there was always the same reaction, always the same reluctance to touch, always the fast withdrawal. I don't know why doctors are so reluctant to carefully touch their patients. Perhaps it is because of their training. Maybe they have been trained to rely on the gadgets they use to examine their patients. Doctors don't realize these gadgets give them, at best, limited information, and, at worst, false information about the cause of their patient's pain.

Take the X-ray, for example. Doctors rely heavily on this device. When someone comes to a doctor complaining of pain, the doctor will carefully study X-rays of **bones** instead of carefully studying the **tissues** of the pain sufferer.

What doctors don't understand is that a person can have an "excellent" X-ray, where nothing dysfunctional shows up, yet suffer severe pain. Or, on the other hand, an X-ray can look "terrible" and the person feels fine. In other words, there is no necessary relationship between an X-ray and the cause of a person's pain. You might discuss this with your doctor the next time she tells you that nothing showed up on your X-ray or advises an operation when something did.

It may be the doctor's training that is behind his reluctance to touch you. It may be the result of an inability to indulge in creative thinking. But even if he had been trained to do so, or had the intelligence to understand that he should do so, your doctor simply doesn't have time to carefully touch you.

I know a doctor who sees forty or more patients a day. I have been told this is not an unusually large workload. I understand that what doctors do nowadays is try to keep four or five examining rooms full at all times and to circulate back and forth as patients are cranked through, one after another. If this is so, what chance does a poor chronic pain sufferer have for a proper examination, not to mention a proper treatment? Very little.

I have not completely given up on trying to find a doctor with whom I can discuss the relationship of pain and soft tissue dysfunction. Not too long ago, a new doctor started a practice in my area. I made an appointment to talk with him. He said he could give me a few moments. I started to describe my approach to treating painful tissue.

He interrupted. "But is it legal?" he asked. I told him of course, it's legal. He said he wasn't sure, and besides, the whole thing sounded "questionable" to him. And then he told me that he had no more time for our visit.

You Are More Than a Collection of Unrelated Anatomical Parts

When patients suffering chronic pain visit doctors, they are not looked upon as unified beings with all parts of their bodies interconnected and interrelated. Doctors look at them, instead, as collections of unrelated anatomical parts. Accordingly, if one part hurts, its pain is thought to be separate, unique, and unrelated to the other parts.

Doctors give names to manifestations of pain. The names spring from where the pain happens to occur. If, at a particular time, pain occurs at the elbow, the doctor's attention is focused there, and the patient is told he has tennis elbow. If, at a particular time, the painful part happens to be a shoulder, attention is directed toward that part of the body, and a name is given for *that* pain. The name may be rotator cuff syndrome. If someone suffers from a painful head, a name is given for that painful area, and the patient is told he has migraine or tension headache.

*Medical "Treatment" for Chronic Pain: Dangerous
Drugs, Mutilating Surgery, and .... Deadening of Nerves.*

Your body, however, is much more than a collection of unrelated body parts. All parts are interconnected and interrelated. If the tissues of one part of your body become dysfunctional, then the rest of your body reacts to that dysfunction. Pain generated by tissue dysfunction inexorably spreads throughout extensive areas of your body and will manifest itself in different parts of your body from time to time. Focusing attention on one area betrays a lack of knowledge of what is causing the pain.

Medical "treatment" of chronic pain is directed toward attempting to reduce pain that flares up here or there as our bodies gradually tighten. Patients are given pain-killing drugs or subjected to surgery directed toward a local symptom of pain, not toward the underlying cause, which is allowed to worsen as the years pass. The tragic result is that countless numbers of people needlessly suffer severe and progressive pain and physical dysfunction for their entire lives.

Your body is much more than a collection of unrelated body parts. All parts are interconnected and interrelated. If the tissues of one part of your body become dysfunctional, then the rest of your body reacts to that dysfunction. Pain generated by tissue dysfunction inexorably spreads throughout extensive areas of your body.

Consider all the individuals who are forced to become residents of nursing homes because their bodies have been allowed to become so stiff and painful that they can no longer take care of themselves, and you will begin to understand the terrible toll society is paying for this medical ignorance.

The Schatz Technique™

Ten Medical Approaches That *Do Not* Reverse Chronic Pain.

Soft tissue has a potential of contracting and pressing on nerves, thus causing the symptoms doctors call "chronic pain." The same tissue also has the potential of having the process reversed and becoming healthy and free of pain--if effective treatment is given. The following are what doctors currently dispense to their pain-suffering patients. Unfortunately, *none of them* will reverse and normalize the contracted tissue that *causes* chronic pain.

1. Dangerous Drugs. *Pain is our friend!* At the present time, doctors consider pain to be our enemy. They should, however, think of pain as a friend, or at least an important messenger. The sensation of pain should be welcomed for what it really is: an alarm signal warning us that our bodies are becoming unhealthy. The focus of treatment shouldn't be to turn off the pain signal. Instead, the focus should be to find what is causing the signal of pain and then to fix that cause. Once the cause is fixed, the pain-alarm goes away and stays away!

When we go to a dentist because of a painful tooth, the dentist does not attempt to overwhelm the alarm signal of pain with dangerous pain-killing drugs. She keeps looking for the source of pain until she finds and fixes it. The pain then goes away, because the problem *causing* the pain has been fixed. Doctors should do what dentists do.

The sensation of pain is necessary for life. Occasionally, someone is born without the ability to perceive pain. The pain sensing apparatus is missing. These unfortunate individuals have a short life span.

They have been denied the warning system that tells the rest of us when something is wrong with our bodies so the problem can be recognized and dealt with. We should learn from this, and, in turn, educate our doctors that the sensation of pain is important and should not be tampered with lightly without inviting dire consequences.

Put it this way: when we hear a fire alarm go off, we realize the fire alarm is our friend. We don't rush over and try to *kill* the fire alarm. *We put out the fire!* Doctors should think about chronic pain the same way the rest of us think about fire alarms.

Pain-killers can kill. Killing the patient's important alarm signal of pain with drugs is bad enough. But those same drugs can actually kill the patient. ALL pain-killing drugs have dangerous side effects. Some can cause you to bleed to death without warning. Others can cause heart attacks, strokes, high blood pressure, and liver and kidney damage. The longer you take these harmful drugs, the greater the chance you will be seriously harmed by them.

These are very real risks. *Thousands* of innocent people die each year because their doctors prescribed these dangerous drugs, and recommended equally dangerous over-the-counter drugs. Did your doctor *carefully* discuss these risks when you were advised to take dangerous drugs?

VIOXX and the August 29, 2000, LARRY KING LIVE SHOW!

Featured guests of the Larry King Live! program of August 29, 2000, included Gold Medal Winners Dorothy Hamill and Bruce Jenner. Hammil and Jenner proudly announced they were now Spokespersons for the drug **VIOXX (remember the Merk Marketing Mantra: "Just One Pill a Day?"**) and were launching their careers that very night! They were then going to tour the country talking about **VIOXX**. The theme of their **VIOXX** campaign, according to Mr. Jenner, was "Everyday Victories."

By becoming Spokespersons for **VIOXX**, Ms. Hamill and Mr. Jenner were linking their names and reputations to a dangerous drug, about which they apparently knew very little. They certainly didn't discuss possible serious side effects of the drug.

Also on the program was Dr. John Klippel, Medical Director of the Arthritis Foundation. He was there to provide the "doctor stuff."

Dr. Klippel spoke favorably about the drug. He did not strongly inform viewers that there were very real and significant risks of bleeding to death, without warning, by taking **VIOXX**. The longer one took the drug, certainly on a daily basis, the greater the danger of death or hospitalization, was not mentioned by Dr. Klippel.

I was astonished that a learned doctor, a rheumatologist, the Medical Director of the Arthritis Foundation, was unaware of these severe risks; and that viewers of the Larry King Live! show were not alerted to them. This alarmed me greatly.

I immediately contacted the Larry King show, presented my credentials and concerns, and suggested that I would be delighted to discuss them with the participants of the program. I am a great fan of Larry King and felt that he would not want to risk the health of his viewers. I received no reply.

I am truly concerned that viewers may have been harmed by what they heard--and didn't hear, on the program. However, my conscience is untroubled because I did all I knew to do to remedy the situation. How others can sleep at night is something I don't understand.

I can understand why I did not receive an answer to my "message of alarm." After all, I was an unknown physical therapist, and these were well known celebrities, and an eminent rheumatology doctor.

....

By the way, Mr. Jenner said on the program: "**we are also doing a lot to support the Arthritis Foundation**."

If what Mr. Jenner said is true, then **Dr. Klippel, who is the Medical Director of the Arthritis Foundation**, should not have been allowed to discuss the drug on the program, because that would have been a clear conflict of interest.

Medical Treatment of Chronic Pain: Dangerous Drugs,
Mutilating Surgery, and .... Deadening of Nerves.

NEWS FLASH!

The FDA, that governmental body assigned to protect us from harmful drugs is in cahoots with the manufacturers of those drugs. The September 25, 2000, issue of USA TODAY, (Volume 19, Number 7, Page 1) presented a banner headline: "FDA advisers tied to the industry." The sub-headline announced: "Drug-approved process riddled with conflicts of interest, analysis finds."

....

It has been nine years since that Larry King Live! program and the USA article appeared. Sad to say, the deep pockets of the Drug Industry have grown ever deeper, and has infiltrated all levels of medical practice. What they tell us, and the doctors that treat us, cannot be trusted. They will say or do anything to sell their drugs, even if they are ineffective or dangerous. And they do it in an extremely sophisticated way, so we are not aware they are behind what is being said.

You might think about that when you are advised to take a pain-killing drug by doctors or celebrities.

2. Mutilating Surgery. Cutting into dysfunctioning tissues with a sharp scalpel *will not normalize them.* Indeed, surgical intrusion causes scar tissues to form, and may damage nerves and blood vessels, thereby complicating the problem. *It's a form of mutilation.*

3. Deadening of Nerves. Attempting to kill the important messenger of pain with drugs, and surgical mutilation of tissues, is inexcusable. But the ultimate insult doctors inflict on their patients is when they *permanently* deaden nerves by cutting them with scalpels, snipping them with scissors, or injecting them with chemicals.

4. Exercise. Regular exercise is necessary for the maintenance of a healthy body. I like to lift weights and perform aerobic workouts. I feel wonderful after these sessions. However, when tight, contracted, fibrotic tissues have developed, stressing those tissues with "forced exercise" as prescribed by doctors, merely stimulates the formation of additional dysfunctioning tissue, thus worsening the condition.

5. Rest. Allowing tight, contracted tissues to "rest" (i.e., moving them as little as possible) may give the body some time to accommodate to the pain of tissue dysfunction. However, the underlying problem remains, and symptoms will reappear when activity is resumed.

6. Stretching. There are two kinds of stretchings: healthy stretching, and unhealthy "forced" stretching as prescribed by doctors. When you yawn and give a pleasant-feeling stretch, that is *healthy* stretching. A cat when it stretches, *that* is healthy stretching! Simply walking about, or getting up from a chair, or putting on clothing--the many hundreds of daily movements we perform without our conscious awareness, gently maintains tissue suppleness. These are all forms of healthy stretching.

Unhealthy stretching occurs when doctors and their assistants use force in an attempt to *instantly* lengthen tissues that have become contracted over a period of years. Forced stretching irritates tissues that are already dysfunctional. Joint movement can be restricted by contracted skin, fascia, ligaments and muscles. For every action there is a reaction: when force is applied to these contracted tissues, their reaction is to tighten even more. The painful act of forced stretching causes tissues to become *increasingly* thickened, fibrotic and painful.

I have treated a number of individuals who participated in sports activities and regularly engaged in stretching programs that *forced* an increase in joint range of motion, yet these people complained of pain throughout their bodies. Examination of their tissues revealed advanced fibrotic development. You might think that constant stretching would cause tissues to become supple and healthy, but this is not the case if the stretching is performed in a forced manner.

If tissues are tight and contracted, they must be gently coaxed to relax and soften; they cannot be forced to relax. Doctors do not understand this when they prescribe stretching and "stretching exercise" for their patients. Attempting to stretch the joints of an elderly person who has accumulated the effects of years of soft tissue dysfunction is painful and unproductive, and yet, sadly, is regularly performed by the medical community.

Elderly individuals frequently fall when the tissues behind their knees get so tight that they cannot straighten them fully when they attempt to stand or walk. This condition allows their legs to buckle without warning, and down they go. The medical approach to this problem is to attempt to forcibly stretch those tight tissues. The falls continue, and it is only a matter of time before a fall fractures an arm or leg.

The tissues throughout the elderly body continue to tighten as the years pass; periodic orders to "stretch the joints" are given, all without result. If the aging individuals survive long enough, eventually their tissues become so tight that they are unable to turn from side to side in bed, and need help even to use a bed pan.

The appropriate treatment for any soft tissue problem is to gently soften and normalize the tight, contracted tissues. When the tight tissues of individuals who fall repeatedly after being subjected to years of painful stretchings are properly treated, the results are rewarding and the falls soon cease.

7. Use of Splints. A splint prevents movement. This "forced rest" may allow the body to temporarily accommodate to an area of tissue dysfunction. However, the dysfunction remains and pain will flare up when movement is resumed.

A word of warning: if your doctor has advised you to wear a splint, such as a "wrist splint" for a *prolonged period*, you need to know that this will likely produce a severe "immobilization problem" that will complicate any condition you already have.

8. Cortisone Injections. Tissue effects are temporary and side effects can be serious.

9. Tens units. These devices attempt to block out the body's alarm signal of pain. They do not eliminate the cause of pain.

10. Visits to Psychiatrists. Pain sufferers are *grossly insulted* when their pain is disbelieved by the people they go to for help (their doctors) and are hustled off to psychiatrists to have their heads examined!

The Problem with Pain "Management"

The present motivation of U.S. "healthcare" is to maximize the efficiency of patient care, to move the patient through the system as efficiently as possible, that is, to spend as little time as possible with the patient.

This is unfortunate for the patient suffering chronic pain. These problems demand appreciable amounts of time, both to investigate the cause and then to treat that cause. The pain patient gets it from both ends. The doctor is too busy to find out what is wrong, and then when the patient is sent out to the rehab center, he is moved through a conveyer-belt system consisting primarily of exercises and stretches, all designed for the practitioner to spend as little hands-on time as possible. When insurance coverage runs out, the patient, as a sort of graduation ritual, is handed a home program of stretches and exercises, and sent on his way.

When patients do not do well, it is made out to be their fault. It is made out that they have not been diligent in doing the exercises and stretches, and therefore are responsible for the lack of improvement whereas, in reality, it is the fault of today's medical system and its practitioners.

The problem with pain management centers is revealed in their title: "management." The motto of pain management centers is: "Give up all hope of having the underlying cause of your chronic pain treated, reversed, and normalized." The assumption and rationale of a pain management center is that those who enter its portals have *already* received appropriate, albeit unsuccessful, treatment for their pain.

Pain management centers have no intention of providing effective treatment for people suffering chronic pain. They merely attempt to "manage" the pain as best they can so the patients can hobble around for the rest of their pain-ridden lives.

I contend there is not now a medical system that provides real treatment for those experiencing chronic pain. If doctors knew how to treat the cause of chronic pain, they would change their pain management centers into pain treatment centers or, better yet, pain *prevention* centers!

Have you made a reservation with your local nursing home? The chances are that you, a member of your family, and friends and acquaintances may end up as residents of a nursing home because of the poor quality of the present "healthcare" system.

When I visit a nursing home, employees come to me and say, "My back (or neck or arms or legs) is killing me, what can I do?" I gently touch the area of pain and am immediately aware how tight, thick, and fibrotic the tissues are.

These are people of all ages and provide a casebook of the progressive effects of soft tissue dysfunction:

- A teenage aide with spasmed neck and back tissues hasn't been to a doctor yet; she merely complains about her pain.

- A nurse in her late twenties goes to a doctor for pain relieving drugs; her tissues are beginning to thicken.

- A certified nursing assistant in her forties hobbles over and shows me her terribly painful knee. I don't have to touch it. I can see the swollen tissues above and below her knee.

  She tells me her doctor has been treating it for a long time with injections. A few months ago, he sent her to an orthopedic surgeon, who did arthroscopic surgery on it that made it worse. She has been going to a physical therapist for several weeks who has her doing exercises and stretches.

  "Bernard," she tells me, "it just kills me to do the things they tell me to do." She shows me how they have her bend her painful knee, and tears come to her eyes. "It hurts so bad, and it gets worse after each treatment. I'm going to stop. I can't take the pain anymore." Her doctor has recently been talking about replacing her knee with a mechanical one.

- A charge nurse in her fifties asks if I will give her back a rub. The tissues of her neck, back, and arms are noticeably thickened, and her

29

head is stooped forward. She demonstrates a pronounced "dowager's hump" (discussed later in this book), a clear sign of significant soft tissue dysfunction. She has given up on doctors and does the best she can with over-the-counter "pain relievers."

• A woman in housekeeping says hello. I ask how her foot is doing. She says it doesn't hurt as much as it did (a surgeon removed a nerve in her foot), but she still gets a lot of pain. "I need to get home as soon as I can and get my foot up because of the pain and swelling," she tells me.

• The head of food service comes up to me. "Bernard," he says, "I need your advice. My whole body is getting tighter. It really worries me. I have a doctor's appointment. What will they do for me?" I look at him and see that his shoulders are pulled forward. His body from his waist up is bent forward. He walks awkwardly, with his knees pointing outward. His entire body is indeed getting tighter.

I tell them all the same thing. They need, and have needed for some time, effective treatments directed toward the areas of their bodies that have become tight and fibrotic. They can still be helped, but there is no system of care that provides effective treatments. It saddens me to tell them this, but it is the truth. They nod their heads in agreement and tell me that what I say makes sense, and then they shuffle off to perform their various duties, pain or no pain.

Shotgun Complaints of Pain and Nerve Damage

When dealing with the medical world, a patient should be cautious these days of complaining about too many areas of pain. There is a good chance she will be hustled off to a psychiatrist.

I was told by a doctor recently that physicians are trained to disbelieve the validity of claims of pain if the complainant mentions more than two or three areas of pain. This is called a "shotgun complaint of pain." The assumption is that the patient has some sort of emotional problem. This doctor disbelieved the pain complaints of a patient he had referred to me.

He told me she was either neurotic or wanted a large compensation award. She had been injured in a car accident eight months earlier and since then had been complaining of severe pain in her neck, chest, both upper extremities, and her upper, mid, and lower back. In his view, these were "shotgun complaints of pain." He didn't believe she was really suffering pain.

What I found when I examined her was extensive areas of severely spasmed and contracted tissue. I could *feel* where her tissues were contracted and spasmed, and could observe her reaction when I touched those areas, so naturally I believed her pain, shotgun or no shotgun.

I wanted her doctor to understand that his patient was experiencing real pain. So I carefully made a chart showing the points of her complaints of pain and how they coincided with the areas of contracted tissue I could feel with my fingers. This would surely demonstrate to the doctor that his patient was experiencing real pain. But when I showed the chart to the good doctor, he looked at me as if I were crazy. I never received another referral from him. By the way, when her case went to court, the doctor stated that he thought her claims of pain were not true.

If doctors properly examined their patients, they would realize that what they have been calling nerve damage is in reality tight, contracted body tissues that press on nerves, thereby generating pain. The problem is with the contracted tissues. When body tissues are properly treated, pressure on nerves is released, and pain goes away.

When a patient complains of severe pain, her doctor may bestow upon the individual the diagnosis of "nerve damage." Frequently (may I say invariably?), this is another case of doctors not understanding their patients' bodies. If doctors properly examined their patients, they would realize that what they have been calling nerve damage is in reality tight, contracted tissues that press on nerves, thereby generating pain. The problem is with the contracted tissues. When tissues are properly treated, pressure on nerves is released, and pain goes away.

31

Doctors do not look beyond the secondary symptom of pain, which they call nerve damage. It is bad enough when doctors dope their patients in an attempt to dull the pain. The ultimate nightmare is when doctors surgically remove (i.e. mutilate) or permanently "deaden" stressed but viable nerve tissue, instead of normalizing the contracted tissue that is causing the problem, thereby allowing the patient to become healthy again. The next time your doctor says you have "nerve damage," ask what he precisely means by that.

How Stress Affects Chronic Pain

There is a lot of talk these days about the painful and unhealthy effects stress has on our bodies. Because doctors do not carefully touch our bodies, they do not understand that the tissues of our bodies change in character when subjected to stress. Therefore, they are unaware that this tissue change ultimately results in pain and a lowered level of health.

For example, I think everyone appreciates that there is a connection between levels of stress and the intensity and frequency of migraine attacks. But doctors think of the relationship of stress and migraine intensity in a vague sort of way. Stress comes our way and the headache, somehow, gets worse.

What is the physical connection between the stress and the headache? Don't bother asking doctors. The primary cause of headaches, tight and contracted tissues, is not understood by the medical community, so what causes migraines to worsen when subjected to increased stress is also not understood.

But you, the reader of this book, now understand the mechanism that causes migraine headaches. You have learned that body tissues contract and tighten around pain receptors when subjected to physical or emotional stress. The squeezed pain receptors send out alarm signals of pain. If these happen to be located in the scalp, neck, and upper back, the resulting pain is called "migraine."

During episodes of increased stress, the pain receptors are squeezed even further, causing the migraine to become more severe and frequent.

This is the connection between migraines and stress. The same dynamic holds true for any chronic pain.

For example, patients frequently experience severe pain in their hip and thigh following hip surgery. It is reasonable to expect pain, even large amounts of pain, following complicated orthopedic procedures. However, the pain I am speaking of is very severe and interferes with rehabilitation, yet it can be effectively treated without high doses of medication.

What happens is that the surgical incision for hip surgery is invariably made through the substance of the tensor fascia lata, a thick band of fascia that extends over the hip joint down to the knee.

The purpose of this structure is to stabilize the hip and knee joints when standing and walking. Throughout the life of an individual, the tensor fascia lata is subjected to a great amount of stress as it performs its important duty. It reacts to this lifetime of stress by becoming tight, contracted, and fibrotic. When a surgeon cuts into this already dysfunctioning tissue, it severely spasms and produces large amounts of pain.

Since orthopedic doctors are not in the habit of carefully examining the soft tissues of their patients, they do not understand that the severe pain their patients experience is not due to the surgical procedure per se, but is caused instead by the reaction of the tensor fascia lata.

When the unfortunate patient complains of excruciating pain and is reluctant to move his leg because of the pain, the doctor either prescribes large amounts of mind-numbing drugs, or, more likely, exhorts the poor soul to "move through the pain." The old, inhumane and counterproductive adage, "no pain, no gain," is still, unfortunately, frequently administered.

The humane and effective approach to this painful situation is to gently explore the tissues of the hip and thigh, so the spasmed area can be located and treated. When spasmed tissues are softened and normalized, pain goes away (it is surprising how comfortable the patient rapidly becomes when properly treated), and the patient begins to move his leg freely. Recovery becomes considerably more rapid.

Ironically, it is a stressed tensor fascia lata that frequently *causes* the hip pain and joint dysfunction that results in surgical intervention, namely, hip joint replacement. This tragically misunderstood and preventable event is discussed later in this book.

The Pain of Misdiagnosed "Obesity"

People with large bulk and heavy weight are thought to be obese; their bulk and weight is attributed to stored fat. I have treated several patients who were described by their doctors as being obese. Some were obese in the stored fat sense; others, however, were different. Their thick, heavy trunks and limbs were thickened by accretions of fibrotic tissue.

The thickened skin of these individuals, when gently palpated, was tender and painful and adherent to underlying tissues. When the underlying tissues were explored, they also revealed themselves to be tender and painful. They were thickened, not by fat, but by fibrotic tissue. The tissues surrounding the joints of these individuals were enlarged, not by accumulations of fat, but by development of thick fibrotic tissue.

These unfortunate individuals were doubly plagued. First, their pain and dysfunction were not appreciated, understood, or properly treated by the medical community. Second, they were described as obese and criticized for being gross overeaters.

Individuals that happen to be obese in the stored fat sense may also suffer soft tissue dysfunction. However, their doctors invariably attribute their pain to their obesity. If someone fails to lose the weight her doctor insists must be lost, the continuing pain is attributed to the continuing obesity. This is duly noted in the individual's medical record and the patient is marked down as being noncompliant (i.e., the patient is at fault, not the doctor). The truth is that the continuing pain is caused by ineffective treatment, not by the obesity.

Pain Disbelieved by Doctors

Most of the patients that come to me with complaints of chronic pain have been disbelieved by their doctors. Many of these pain sufferers made the rounds from general practitioner, neurologist, orthopedist, psychiatrist, and back to the general practitioner. After all the medical treatments had been administered and they continued to complain of pain, their doctors had two choices:

1. They could believe their patients were really experiencing pain (which would mean they hadn't known how to properly treat them).

2. They could disbelieve their patients' complaints of pain.

Their doctors chose to disbelieve them. Suffering pain was bad enough, but what made it particularly galling for these pain sufferers was being disbelieved by the very people to whom they had gone for help.

One woman told me she hoped her doctors had found cancer. "At least they would have believed me," she said. Another woman spoke of a similar hope but this time with HIV. Both of these women and many others were relieved when I told them I believed they were having pain and pointed out the cause of their pain. They were pleased when their pain and other symptoms began to diminish, and they were elated when they became pain-free and healthy again.

The Pain Patient's Bill of Rights

I close this chapter on pain with a declaration that I call "The Pain Patient's Bill of Rights."
 • It is our right to live without chronic pain. It is the obligation of our doctors to see that right attained and to pursue that right with diligence, enthusiasm, dedication, and intelligence.
 • It is our right to be believed, and to be treated with dignity and respect when we say we are experiencing pain. We will not allow our pain to be trivialized, dismissed, or not addressed at all. We will refuse to go to psychiatrists simply because our doctors do not have the necessary knowledge or compassion to realize we really are suffering pain.
 • We demand that doctors acknowledge that pain is an alarm, warning us that something in our bodies is not working

properly, and stop dosing us with pain killers designed to turn off the important alarm signal; that pain is merely a symptom, not the cause of body dysfunction; and since doctors have assumed total responsibility for the care of our bodies, that they fix the cause so the symptom of pain will go away and we will become healthy again.

- It is our right to receive a thorough, intensive, and appropriate examination to determine the cause of our pain, however much examination time that may take. We will not accept one that is hurried and cursory and rushes us through as quickly as possible. It is the doctors themselves that set up the system of healthcare now in place, so they do not have the right to say they do not have the time to properly examine us.

- We demand that doctors carefully examine our bodies, carefully touch our bodies so they will understand how our bodies have changed and how this change is the cause of our pain. If doctors are unwilling or unable to determine the underlying dysfunction that is causing our pain, we demand that they acknowledge their ignorance instead of pretending expertise and implying knowledge.

- We will not accept the onus and responsibility for our continued pain. The inappropriate, misguided, and ineffective care our doctors have been providing should be faulted, not us.

- We will strongly question the proposition that our pain is irreversible, that nothing more can be done. We understand that if we are told this, the people saying it probably do not know what is causing our pain or how to treat it.

- We demand that a system of care be designed and implemented that will treat the underlying cause of our pain and diminished health, not the present one that deals only with secondary symptoms.

- **We, the patients suffering chronic pain, will no longer tolerate a system that tells us to endure pain for the rest of our lives.**

The Schatz Technique™
Brand Pain Prevention *and* Treatment Method:

Real Treatment of Chronic Pain

The reality of your body and the pain that it holds, is the end result of a *process* that has developed over your lifetime. It is necessary to reverse that process if your body is to become healthy and pain-free once again. The gentle persuasion of *The Schatz Technique™* does just that... and this is the very essence of real treatment for chronic pain: *the reversal of the process!*

I have studied and treated soft tissue dysfunction for over fifty years, and have been a sculptor for the same period of time. In my approach to treating soft tissue dysfunction, the primary *cause* of chronic pain, I combine the skills I developed as a sculptor, using my fingers that shape clay to also shape body tissue, together with the discoveries gained in my half-century study of tissue dysfunction. I call the technique I originated *"The Schatz Technique™ ."*

In order to provide real and lasting treatment to those who suffer chronic pain, the tissue systems of skin, fascia, muscles, and ligaments have to be carefully examined and normalized when dysfunction is found. That is to say, each tissue system has to be treated. Osteopaths and chiropractors manipulate vertebrae of the spinal column. I have discovered how to release contracted tissue, and I will now pass this knowledge on to you.

The Schatz Technique ™ Brand Pain Prevention *and* Treatment Method Is Different from Massage

I have great respect for those who do massage. They use their hands to help their clients, and I applaud what they do, but we do different things.

The Schatz Technique™

I use my fingers to carefully *explore* and release specific tissue systems. For example, I may choose during a particular treatment session to work on only the skin, or muscle tissue, or fascia, or ligaments. Perhaps in a session I may treat all those tissues, but treatment of tissue dysfunction is only effective if each tissue system is treated thoroughly.

I apply my techniques directly to a specific area of tissue dysfunction and work on that particular area until it softens and becomes healthy again. If I have to work on a small area of the palm of a hand for an entire two-hour session in order to soften and heal the tissues overlying the carpal tunnel, then that is what I will do.

People who do massage are oriented to work in a more general manner, to work on the body as a whole in a particular session. And the effects they obtain can be wonderful. Clients leave their massage tables relaxed and with a sense of well-being.

Let me put it this way. From time to time, I have traded sessions with persons who do massage. I expect treating fingers to look for specific areas of tissue dysfunction, and this does not happen. True, after the session I feel relaxed overall. But I await exploration and treatment if dysfunction is found, and this does not occur. Conversely, I cannot perform the broad movements they expect. My fingers continually pause in their search for specific areas of tissue dysfunction.

This section presents an overview of *The Schatz Technique™* . The following section will describe the technique in great detail, so you can treat your chronic pain.

When I treat someone who suffers shoulder, arm, head, hand, back, or leg pain, I don't care what catchy name doctors have given that pain. It doesn't matter if he has called it migraine, carpal tunnel syndrome, or thingamabob. The treatment approach is the same wherever the cause of pain occurs:

1. Locate the dysfunctioning tissues that are squeezing pain receptors, and
2. Normalize those dysfunctioning tissues, thereby releasing the pain receptors so the pain will go away and the body can become healthy.

When my fingers find tissues that have grown tight, thick, hard, and painful, I gently apply the technique to coax the tissues to soften and become painless.

I work with clay in much the same way. When sculpting, I gently coax the clay into the form that is in my mind. Clay cannot be forced into a different shape; it must be coaxed. So it is with body tissues: they cannot be forced into a healthier form; they too must be gently coaxed.

Tight, contracted, fibrotic body tissues will succumb to gentle persuasion. One can be gentle and still be profoundly effective. However, treatment must be directed to specific tissue dysfunction. When this is done, the results can be astonishing.

The Connecting Agent: How to Discover the

Pain's Source

In order to locate dysfunctioning tissues that squeeze pain receptors, the fingers must be intimately connected with those tissues; a connecting agent must be used. I made this important discovery several years ago.

Doctors use a connecting agent (they call it a coupling agent) when they look inside bodies with ultrasound. Without a connecting agent, gel or lotion, the ultrasound sees nothing; it is blind. Unfortunately, ultrasound cannot "see" soft tissue dysfunction. Fingers must "feel" tissue dysfunction. And they are blind to the feel of dysfunctioning tissues if they do not have a connecting agent to find the "enemy," the thick, fibrotic tissue. Invariably, the patient says, "Yes, that's just where I hurt!" Examining a patient's body without the use of a connecting agent is like the blind trying to read without the use of Braille.

In the future, when patients with chronic pain go to practitioners for help, their practitioners will carefully examine their entire body. With the use of a connecting or discovering agent, all will be known so proper treatment can be directed to dysfunctioning tissues. **When people get periodic tissue checks and treatments early on, pain and physical dysfunction will be prevented.**

Overview of *The Schatz Technique™*
Brand Pain Prevention *and* Treatment Method

To reverse severe soft tissue dysfunction, treatment must be <u>specifically directed to the dysfunctioning tissue</u>. Although soft tissue dysfunction tends to be global in nature (that is, large areas of the body are affected), the severity of dysfunction varies from place to place, and from tissue system to tissue system (skin, muscle, fascia, ligament).

Let us say that we are treating the tissues of a painful left shoulder blade. (I selected the shoulder blade as an example of treatment because I once treated someone whose shoulder blade was crisscrossed with surgical scars inflicted in misguided and failed attempts to surgically correct a soft tissue problem). Some areas of the skin overlying the shoulder blade are severely tight, thick, and adherent to underlying tissues. Other areas are similarly affected, but less so. Still others are not affected at all. The unhealthy areas of skin have to be located, discovered with a connecting agent, in order for them to be treated.

The same is true for the other tissue systems of that area. We need to identify dysfunctioning portions of the muscules that connect the shoulder blade to the spinal column, as well as other areas of muscules that might be involved. **Dysfunctioning skin, muscles, fascia and ligaments have to be identified so they can be treated and normalized, thereby releasing their tight hold on pain receptors.** *The body will then become healthy and free of pain.*

40

The first step of treatment is to *touch* the patient's body. This simple but important act begins the process that enables the practitioner's fingers to find those tight, thick, unhealthy tissues.

We have the patient with left shoulder blade pain lying on his *left* side (unless this position is uncomfortable). This position approximates (brings closer together) that shoulder blade and the spinal column, thus providing some slack in the tissues and making them more easily investigated. I apply some lotion to the area of skin between the shoulder blade and the spinal column. I move my fingers in a variety of exploratory movements, up and down, in circles, and back and forth.

> *The first step of treatment is to touch the patient's body. This simple but important act begins the process that enables the practitioner's fingers to find those tight, thick, unhealthy tissues.*

My fingers are now concentrating on the skin. They are looking for hard, thick, or lumpy areas. *There's* an area that's thick. I make a mental note of it and will come back later to soften and release it. As I find other areas that need treatment, I note where they are located.

The lotion is drying out, causing my fingers to drag, so I add a bit more. My fingers move smoothly over the skin again. I ripple portions of the skin gently between my thumb and fingers; this gives additional information. I find areas that become painful after a bit of gentle investigation. These are hidden pain areas, they tell me these areas need treatment. I continue working, moving out to the shoulder blade proper.

I add a few drops of water to the lotioned skin. This provides a different connecting effect. It allows my fingers to glide over the skin just a bit differently so additional information can be elicited.

When I feel this mode of investigation has yielded an appropriate amount of information, I wipe off the lotion. I can now grasp small portions of the skin and move them over the underlying tissues. Trying small back-and-forth and circling movements, I find areas of skin that won't glide over the tissues under it because they are "stuck" to the tissues underneath. Adherent skin indicates severe dysfunction of tissues deeper in the body. So I always examine the skin carefully.

Reapplying lotion, I turn my attention to the deeper tissues, using my fingertips on the surface of the skin to gently probe and nudge the tissues underlying the skin. It is surprising how much information can be obtained this way about the condition of deep tissues. My fingers look for tight, thick musculature, fascia, and ligaments. They search for fibrotic configurations. I note anything that is not soft and supple. I ask the patient to let me know if I touch anything that is tender or painful. I note where these places are.

When I have thoroughly examined the deeper tissues, I have the patient turn onto his right side. Every examining position yields particular and unique information, although I rarely have the patient lie facedown, because this position is usually uncomfortable and tends to stretch the tissues of the back, making them difficult to palpate and treat. I explore the skin and deeper tissues from this position. Now that the shoulder is upwards, I can hold and gently move it with my left hand while with my right hand I examine the tissues that are being moved about. This gives me additional important information.

I then have the patient turn so he is lying on his back, and follow the same procedures. Gently slipping the fingers under a lotioned back in this position can yield abundant tissue information. When I have examined the skin and underlying tissues, I am ready to use the information to plan my treatment approach.

Now begins the normalizing phase of treatment. There are few things more exciting to me than locating tight, dysfunctioning body tissues that are causing severe pain, and then to release those tissues and hear the patient say that the pain is gone. Lotion, essential as a connecting or discovering agent in the examining phase, is equally important in the normalizing phase, for without it *The Schatz Technique™* cannot be directed to specific areas of tissue dysfunction.

I often start treatment by softening the skin. So, when working on that shoulder blade, I begin by applying lotion and rippling the skin bordering the spinal column at the level of the low back, and moving gently upward.

All goes smoothly until I encounter one of the areas located earlier. Here, I feel the skin is thicker, so I slow down and become even gentler. At the same time, the patient reports there is pain at that spot. I try a few more rippling movements, but the thickness proves to be stubborn, so I back off and try a different method. This time, my fingers perform small, nudging movements that gently coax the stubborn area to let go. Success is achieved: The area softens, the pain goes away, and I move on.

I go back to the rippling movement. When I find other areas that are thick and painful, I pause and try to coax them to let go, to soften. With some, I am successful; with others, I will have to return at a future session when I can spend more time on them.

As treatment continues, I use a variety of movements. The greater the variety of movements used, the better the result--not only for treating the skin, but for the treatment of all tissue systems. On certain areas, I use an abundant amount of lotion; on others, a scant amount. On still others, I use water with just a bit of lotion in it. Constant variation to suit the particular situation encountered is part of the secret of success. The surprising thing is that success is usually achieved. Most of the patients I work with have been told by their doctors that they will live in pain for the rest of their lives. Their problems are extremely severe and complicated, and yet they respond surprisingly well to gentle treatment, and their pain subsides as their tissues become healthy.

When the skin has been appropriately dealt with, I turn my attention to the deeper tissues and structures. One of the techniques I use to release tissues lying deep within the body is difficult to describe, but I will try. Picture a loaf of bread. In the center of the loaf you have (somehow) placed a banana. Hold the loaf in both hands and gently press and release the surface of the loaf. You are creating pulsating waves that go deep and wash over the banana. So it is with the body. By gentle movements at the surface, tissues deep down can be powerfully affected.

Another technique to reach deep tissues is a variation of the nudging movement used to examine body tissues. When my fingers revisit the deep dysfunctioning tissues identified earlier, I gently nudge and coax them to relax and soften. I take as much time as necessary to do this. One cannot coax and rush at the same time.

I will use the wave variations, the nudgings, and other movements to coax the tissues of the shoulder blade and its adjacent tissues to become softened and normalized. I treat the patient while he lies on his right and left sides and face-up to gain every advantage the different approaches afford. By this time, the patient is very likely to say, "Boy, that feels a lot better!"

The degree to which you are successful in reversing tight, contracted, and fibrotic tissue and eliminating pain depends largely on two things: how severe the physical injury or emotional trauma was, and how long the time interval between the onset of injury or trauma and when effective treatment is started.

I have treated more than one individual who was severely injured in early youth, at four or five years of age, and whose treatment, directed toward reducing and reversing the tight, contracted, fibrotic tissue, was not started until they were in their forties, fifties, sixties, or even older. In these individuals, dramatic improvement is still likely, although complete normalization is not. For others, who developed soft tissue dysfunction over their lifetime but who did not suffer severe injury or trauma, treatment is likely to achieve a near-normal result.

If treatment is started four, five, or six years following onset of the problem, then complete reversal is the probable outcome. If effective treatment is started within weeks or months of onset, before the establishment of extensive tissue dysfunction, then the expectation for complete reversal is even better. But even with the worst case scenario, significant reduction of pain and physical dysfunction can be expected.

The Schatz Technique™ Brand Pain Prevention *and* Treatment Method
You Can Treat Yourself: Using Your Fingers Like Eyes

You will now learn how you can treat the cause of your pain. You will get connected with your body and learn a lot about it. I think you will find it interesting and exciting. I know you will be thrilled and delighted when your pain goes away and your body becomes healthy again.

Soft tissue dysfunction underlies the pain to which doctors have affixed various names related to *where* in the body the dysfunction happens to occur. In the remainder of the book, I will discuss some of them and present case histories that illustrate the results of real treatment.

Following each case history, I will present elements of *The Schatz Technique™* you can use on yourself if you have a similar problem.

The human species has an inherent tendency to "rub" an area of pain--the part of our body that is hurting. Rubbing might make the part feel a little better at the time but it does not normalize tissues. I refer to rubbing as the "R" word.

There is another word I refer to with a single letter, and that is the "M" word. "M" stands for massage. "M" and "R" words are not part of the Schatz Technique. The word to use is "explore."

So:

1. We do NOT rub tissues (the "R" word).

2. We do NOT massage tissues (the"M" word).

3. We DO <u>explore</u> tissues.

In order to perform the Schatz Technique it is necessary to overcome the habit of rubbing or massaging and replace it with the act of exploring--indeed, it is essential to do so. Here is what I tell beginners. (Read the following carefully, it is very important):

Don't try to make an area feel better. If you try to make an area feel better (i.e., to instantly change the condition of the tissues) you fall into the trap of repetitious and unproductive rubbing/massaging. Merely *explore* the painful area. Trying to make things better inevitably leads to R and M which does not heal tissues. Gentle exploring provides <u>just the right amount</u> of pressure to heal painful tissues. The more you explore, the greater the amount of healing. Beginners need to forget about changing things---just explore!

Think of it this way: when you rub or massage, you are forcing something *onto* tissues, whether they (the poor, innocent, suffering tissues) like it or not. However, when you gently explore those tissues, you allow them the opportunity of telling you what they want and need and how much. Rubbing and massaging is intruding on the tissues, it's like shoving yourself through a doorway without being invited.

Here is something that will help to eradicate the habit of repetitious rubbing/massaging: Perform <u>only</u> three exploring movements at a time. That is to say, make three gentle circles with your fingers, then stop! After a short pause, make three more exploring movements, stop! Pause, three movements, stop! Pause, three movements.... And so on.

This procedure will not only help break the habit of non-exploring R and M, it will also assist you to develop a sense of patience, of taking your time, rather than rushing through a treatment session. And, the pauses help your fingers educate themselves to the variations of tissue textures by giving them time to process the information coming into them. As experience builds, the exploring movements will become continuous, without the intermediate pauses.

However, always be on guard of the danger of unfocused repetitious rubbing/massaging sneaking up on you unnoticed. Even I, who have been treating for so many years, might find myself, if I get distracted, look down and see that my fingers have stopped exploring and instead are repetitiously massaging or rubbing.

I would like to say something at this point about massage and massage therapists. Massage therapists are intelligent and dedicated to help their clients--and their clients do feel wonderful after a massage. I intend no criticism of them. But, as indicated above and earlier in the book, we do different things. However, since massage therapists are intelligent they certainly can learn to incorporate elements of the Schatz Technique into their practice if they choose to do so.

Before you treat your body, a few basic ideas need to be mentioned:

1. The heart of the Schatz Technique is to gently explore your tissues. Everything flows from this. People are astonished that gentle can be powerful--but it is so. Think of your fingers as having eyes. This may help you "get" the concept of exploring tissues.

2. The part of the body being treated must be as relaxed and comfortable as possible. For example, if you are treating an arm, rest it on a pillow; don't hold it upright. Change positions as often as necessary to stay comfortable and avoid any strain to the body.

3. The use of lotion (oils don't work) as a connecting and exploring agent is essential for reasons mentioned earlier. Unfortunately, most lotions on the market contain large amounts of oil, glycerin or similar products that make them uncontrollably slippery for proper treatment. Look for a lotion that develops a bit of friction as it dries. A little more lotion, or a drop or two of water can be added, to get just the

amount of slipperiness desired. I have developed a lotion that suits the needs of *The Schatz Technique™* . It is available on my website.

4. Fingernails must be closely trimmed. You will be using your fingertips as well as the pads of your fingers.

5. When you work on tissue that is very hard and fibrotic, become particularly gentle.

6. Think of what you are doing as an exciting adventure. I feel confident that when the tissues of your body respond and become healthy and free of pain, you will indeed be thrilled.

7. It may take a session or two before your fingers are able to sense the soft tissue dysfunction that underlies your chronic pain. I gradually developed an appreciation of how tissues feel when they become tight and contracted. This book gives you the advantage of knowing what to look for before you start.

8. Keep in mind that the whole process is simple. You apply lotion to a part of your body that is painful, and your fingers look for tight, contracted tissues. You perform exploring movements, the process reverses and pain and tightness go away.

Instructions for *The Schatz Technique™* may appear to be complicated at first glance, much as instructions for assembling a bookcase may look complicated. But once you try, you will find they are simple and easy to follow. I suggest that you tape-record the treatment instructions for your area of pain so you can listen to them as you do the movements.

9. Set aside as much time that you have available for self-treatment of your chronic pain--the more time, the better. If you only have 15 minutes--that will do to get things started. 30 minute sessions would be even better. Each session has a cumulative effective--your body will become healthier and healthier.

It is very likely that you will become so absorbed with the excitement of the process that when you glance at the clock you will be amazed at how much time has flown by!

10. Before you treat yourself, review the glossary to get acquainted with technique terminology. Look over the anatomical landmark drawings as well. Don't feel you have to memorize them; they are meant only to be helpful. Soft tissue treatment is an exciting, creative experience. It is not a boring, rigid "cookbook" routine. Early on, it would be wise to closely follow treatment suggestions. However, once you gain experience, feel free to experiment. After all, every time I treat, I learn a bit more.

I wish you the very best and hope you have the greatest success in helping yourself to become healthy and pain-free!

Frequently Asked Questions

Readers, even when their bodies improve and their pain lessens, ask: **"How do I know what to look for?" "How do I know I am finding the right things?"**

The answer is simple-- it is all so simple that sometimes beginners have difficulty wrapping their mnds around the simplicity of it. The body is so complex, I don't fully understand the dynamics of it. However, something wonderful happens when your fingers simply **explore** your tissues!

You don't have to "look for things" or "find things." Just explore! That is to say: **get acquainted with the tissues of your body!** The simple act of exploring, in itself, initiates the healing process. The more time you spend "exploring," the more your fingers will become "educated" and you will begin to "find things." Even before this happens, your body will begin to heal if you just relax and simply explore.

If you do have any remaining questions, feel free to contact me at:

Bernard@ReverseYourPain.com

PART TWO:

How You Can
Treat Your Own Pain

The Schatz Technique™
Brand Pain Prevention *and* Treatment Method
Glossary of Terms

Please do not think of the following technique terms as massage movements that are *imposed* on the body. Rather, think of them as a variety of gentle methods of "exploring" the tissues of the body–of using your fingers like eyes.

Back-and-forths: Particularly helpful in tracking and treating long, narrow bands of dysfunctioning tissue. Place one or more fingers at an area of dysfunction; move them back and forth in one-inch travels.

Circles: Thumb, single finger, or multiple fingers are used to make small or large circles. This is for exploring and treating skin or underlying tissues.

Drags: The pads of fingers or thumb are brought against unlotioned or lightly lotioned skin. This movement is similar to sweeps, but firmer, for deeper tissue.

Floats: A liberal amount of lotion is applied to the skin and diluted with a few drops of water. This allows one or more fingers to float easily over the surface of the skin. Minute patterns of fibrotic configurations can be detected in this manner. It also allows very painful areas to be treated very gently.

Jiggling: The pads of the outstretched fingers are placed against the target tissue. The distal finger joints are rapidly flexed and straightened, causing the tissues to jiggle. This gentle treatment technique creates powerful movement of large areas of tissues. It is very effective at the forearm and calves.

Kneading: This exploring movement is similar to kneading bread or pastry.

Nudging: This technique is used to normalize well-defined areas of tissue dysfunction, and thumb or fingers can be used. Approach the border of the target tissue and direct the movement toward its center. Imagine a raisin glued to a tabletop. You want to soften that raisin as much as possible, so you gently and patiently nudge it from all directions.

Palming: The palm is placed closely against the skin of the target area and moved in circles or back-and-forths. This technique is frequently used on unlotioned skin as a means of loosening adherent bonds.

Planing: The fingers and palm are held flat against the skin. Used in a similar fashion as a carpenter's plane to shave outer layers of wood. The technique is applied when lotion has dried to provide gentle friction. Try with fingers leading the movement, then after a time, use variation of back and forths–fingers lead, then backing up with palm leading in the opposite direction (fingers-palm, palm-fingers...). Planing is useful in reducing skin thickness and improving body contours.

Probes: The tip of a single finger is used to explore deeper tissues.

Push-pulls: This is one of the movements of pincering. The tissue is between the thumb and forefinger. The thumb pushes the tissue against the forefinger; the forefinger then pushes the tissue back against the thumb so that the tissue is pushed and pulled, effectively used at the web of the thumb, for example.

Shaking: This can be used at a joint or with a broad area of tissue. Pincer the joint or tissue between the thumb and forefinger, and gently shake. This movement is particularly useful with tissue configurations such as the biceps, or thumb and finger joints.

Skin Grasping: This is used to free a local area of adherent skin from underlying tissues. Grasp a small bit of skin between thumb and forefinger; move it in small circles and back-and-forths.

Skin Rippling: This technique is used to identify and normalize (1) thickened, fibrotic areas of the skin, (2) hidden pain areas, and (3) areas of the skin that are adherent to underlying tissue. Place thumb and fingers on the skin; move the thumb toward fingers. As this is performed, allow the skin to move wavelike under the advancing thumb. Thick, adherent skin will not ripple.

Stationary Pressing: A single finger, multiple fingers, or the thumb can be used to press gently but firmly on a tissue area. This is useful for treating severely painful areas, where movement would be uncomfortable, and it's useful in softening creases.

Sweeps: The flat edge of the thumb, single finger, or multiple fingers are used in sweeping motions, as if you were smoothing down the hair of your forearm, or brushing crumbs off a tabletop. This is useful for gently treating the skin.

Waves: Here, wavelike patterns go down into deep tissues. These are set up at the surface of the body by gentle pulsating movements of the palms or finger pads.

Anatomical Landmarks

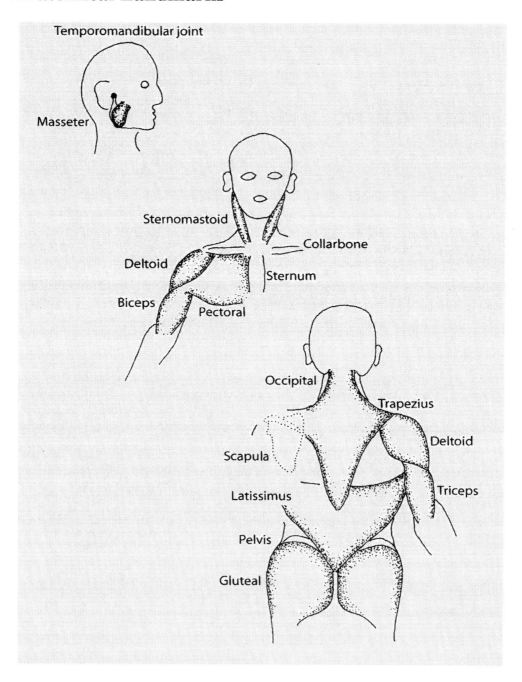

Arthritis

Did your doctor tell you that your pain is caused by arthritis?

Question: did your doctor carefully examine your *tissues*, to see if soft tissue dysfunction is the cause of your pain? Tissue dysfunction can produce the symptoms of arthritis. **If your tissues were not carefully examined, you did not receive a proper examination.**

The word "arthritis" has lost almost all of its meaning these days. In the old days, arthritis meant an inflamed joint ("arthro"=joint, "itis"=inflammation). Nowadays doctors call *any* ache or pain "arthritis."

Doctors tell us that "osteoarthritis" is the most common form of arthritis. However, what they are referring to is a *degenerative* process of cartilage. A degenerative process is NOT an inflammatory process. So, why take expensive and dangerous anti-inflammatory drugs for this non-inflammatory condition? Indeed, the use of these drugs can actually *damage* cartilage.

As mentioned throughout this book, doctors do not know how to examine patients suffering chronic pain. They therefore do not realize that the pain and stiffness affecting so many millions, that they have been *calling* osteoarthritis, is *really* soft tissue dysfunction occurring outside innocent joints.

There are some doctors who are more creative in the names they invent for so-called arthritis. Take the following case, for example.

Case History

A printer who heard of my work had obtained a referral from his physician and arranged for an appointment. He had been treated for several years by an arthritis specialist for what the "specialist" called "serum negative" arthritis. The printer suffered severe pain throughout his body. The pain was constant with episodes of exacerbated, unbearable pain.

The problem had started seventeen years earlier after he injured his back in a fall. Gradually, over the years, the pain spread from his back to all parts of his body, including his arms and legs. The arthritis specialist had treated him with various medications and pain-killers, but his symptoms had steadily worsened, and the frequency and intensity of the flare-ups had recently increased.

At the time of our first treatment, the pain in his hands was so severe that he could only use them as "paddles," with fingers outstretched. He was greatly concerned that, because of his inability to use his hands properly, he was about to lose his job.

When I examined his body, I found that all of his tissues were tight, contracted, and extremely painful, from the top of his scalp to the soles of his feet. But at the end of the first treatment, he stated that his pain was down seventy-five percent. He could use his hands in a near-normal fashion. He was delighted.

I continued to work with him for two months. He was then free of any pain and could perform his job without any problem.

He called a few months later to report a flare-up of pain, and returned for a few more treatments. The flare-up coincided with a stressful marital problem. I continued to see him every three or four months for flare-ups that coincided with marital-stress episodes. These flare-ups responded favorably to one to three treatments.

56

Two years after I had first seen him, he called to say that he and his wife had separated and that he was leaving the area. He thanked me for the help I had given him and said he was feeling fine.

This person had suffered severe pain and physical dysfunction for several years because of the inability of his doctor to understand what his problem was and how to properly treat it. He had been given various arthritis and pain "medications," all to no avail.

We found, however, that his pain was caused by tight, contracted tissues that squeezed pain receptors. When I released the contracted tissues surrounding his pain receptors, his pain went away. During the episodes of marital stress, his body tissues retightened, again squeezing the pain receptors located within them.

The tissue systems of our body, primarily the skin, muscles, fascia, and ligaments, respond to physical and emotional insults by contracting. In other words, both emotional and physical stress can cause soft tissue dysfunction that results in pain.

As mentioned earlier in this book, the tissue systems of our body, primarily the skin, muscles, fascia, and ligaments, respond to physical and emotional insults by contracting. In other words, both emotional and physical stress can cause soft tissue dysfunction that results in pain. Emotional stress was an important factor of this individual's soft tissue pain that was misdiagnosed as arthritis pain.

The Schatz Technique™ Instructions

Soft tissue dysfunction that is misdiagnosed as arthritis can occur anywhere on your body. I suggest you start by examining and treating your arms, hips, and knees. Refer to "Carpal Tunnel Syndrome," "Hip Pain and Degenerative Joint Disease," and "Knee Pain" for *The Schatz Technique*™ instructions.

Back Pain

X-rays, MRI's, and CAT scans identify the cause of only a small percentage of back pain. Did you know that the cause of over 80 percent of back pain remains unaccounted for by doctors? They will continue to be baffled by back pain until they learn to carefully touch their patients.

I have observed all kinds of medical "treatments" that are directed toward back pain, going back fifty years to when I was involved in research at Cedars of Lebanon Hospital in Los Angeles in 1950. I have studied the consequences of mutilating surgeries, as well as the poor results of traction devices, medications and modalities such as exercise, stretches, and ultrasound.

Over the years, numerous medical innovations, some of them so-called high tech, have been introduced. In one large facility, I saw physical therapists tightly strap sufferers of severe back pain into cages controlled by computers. The victims were exhorted to push, bend, and twist their painful backs with all their might against the force of their computer-driven cages. If they refused or did not push mightily enough, no matter how severe the pain, negative notations were entered into their charts, and they were branded as malingerers.

Case History 1

A young woman was referred to me because she had been experiencing severe back pain that had been progressing over a period of two years. At first, the pain had been mild and intermittent, but as the months went by, the pain had become increasingly severe and constant. She had been given muscle relaxants, pain medication, and stretching exercises, but the pain continued to worsen.

When I examined her, I found that the tissues of her middle to lower back were tight and contracted, and in addition the tissues of her right gluteal area were tight, contracted, fibrotic, and painful to mild examination. At first, she responded rapidly to treatment. Within two weeks, she had minimal, infrequent pain. But then her improvement slowed. I continued to treat her twice a week for one month, but her remaining pain stubbornly resisted treatment.

At that point, I found something interesting: a small, hard "knot" of tissue in her right gluteal area. I concentrated my efforts on reducing the knot and, as it softened, her remaining pain rapidly cleared.

Just before she was discharged from treatment, she recalled that she had been given a penicillin injection in exactly that spot a month or two before she began experiencing her back pain. Apparently, the penicillin had irritated tissues at the injection site, causing them to spasm, contract, and become fibrotic. Gradually this area had triggered other areas to contract and become painful. The result eventually was the severe and continuous pain she was experiencing when she came for treatment.

It is highly unlikely that the sequence of events that led to this woman's back pain would have been unraveled unless someone had taken the time to carefully examine and treat her. She would have been added to the millions who needlessly suffer severe pain for the entirety of their lives.

Case History 2

A patient was referred because of back pain that had persisted and progressed over a thirty-year period. He had injured his back in his teens when he attempted to lift a heavy weight.

At the time of the injury, he experienced severe, painful spasm of his low back. Pain radiated down both legs. His doctor admitted him to a hospital, where he was placed in continuous traction and was given strong pain medication. Following his discharge from the hospital, his symptoms gradually eased, but he was "never the same" after this.

From time to time, he had flare-ups of pain of varying intensity. He could go for weeks or months with little or no pain, but was always aware that his low back was his problem area and that if he was not extremely careful, the pain in his back would flare up intensely. Or he might go for long periods of time with little or no pain, when for no reason he would have a flare-up of severe, excruciating pain, accompanied by intense spasming and tightening of the tissues of his lower back, incapacitating him for one or two weeks. He was given anti-inflammatory drugs, muscle relaxants, and pain relievers when these flare-ups occurred, which helped to take the edge off the severity of pain.

As the years passed, he noticed that the episodes of pain were becoming more frequent and intense and were lasting longer. By the time he came to see me, his life had become one long, continuous misery.

When I examined him, I found that the tissues of his entire back, particularly from his middle to lower back, down to his gluteals, were tight, contracted, and severely fibrotic, and tender to light touch. Thick, tough, fibrotic bands around the brim of his pelvis were easily palpated. The skin overlying these areas was thick, adherent to substructures, and was very tender to light touch.

The severity of his pain began to subside early in treatment. However, the thick, fibrotic tissues were slow to respond. By the end of three months of treatment, he was free of pain, although appreciable amounts of the thick, fibrotic bands that had developed over the years remained.

Occasionally, he felt that his back was retightening. At those times, he called for an appointment, and we resoftened the tissues that had begun to tighten again. I kept him pain-free over a four year period, but after that I lost track of him.

The Schatz Technique™ Instructions

Soft tissue dysfunction of the upper, middle, and lower back, as well as tissues of the gluteal region, can contribute to back pain. All these areas will require investigation and possible treatment. It may be challenging for you to treat those areas, but it can be done. I know because I successfully self-treated *my* chronic back pain several years ago.

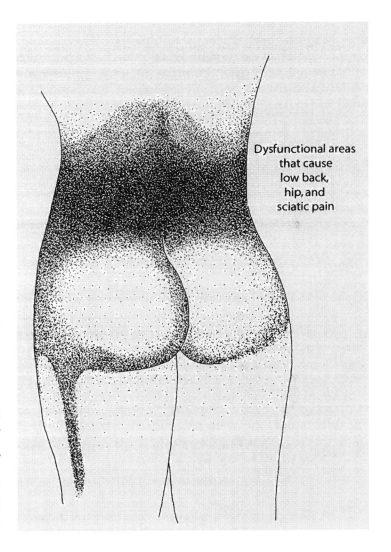

Dysfunctional areas that cause low back, hip, and sciatic pain

Treat yourself while you lie on your side, first one side, then the other. Lying face down stretches the tissues of the back and makes it difficult to work on them. I suggest that you lie on a sofa with your back facing the back of the sofa, but a few inches away from it. This allows you to lean the elbow of your treating hand against the sofa during treatment, thereby reducing fatigue and providing leverage.

Place one or more pillows between your legs. This will not only make your knees more comfortable, but, even more importantly, will put some slack in the uppermost thigh and gluteal tissues, making their treatment more effective. I suggest that you cover the sofa with a sheet and some towels; the chances are that some lotion will drip on them. Have your lotion and a cup of warm water close by.

This first treatment will be a "get acquainted with your body" session. Relax, you have a lot of work ahead of you. Pace yourself; don't try to get it done all at once.

Let's say that you are lying first on your left side. Reach back with your right hand and run it over your back and gluteal areas.

Do this first without lotion, to get a preliminary feel of things. Reach up as high as you can in the direction of your head. Go down to the gluteal area. Bend your knees toward your chest and see how that stretches the gluteal tissues. This makes it difficult to treat them. You will treat the gluteal tissues with your hips and knees comfortably straight.

Apply some lotion to your back. Start up as high as you can reach. With multiple-finger back-and-forths, follow the muscles that run along the side of your backbone. Use the knuckles of your fingers, then the pads of your outstretched fingers. Alternate this throughout the treatment to avoid fatigue.

Go down as far as your pelvis. While you are there, preliminarily explore the brim of your pelvis with thumb circles and back-and-forths. Look for fibrotic thickenings that are adherent to your pelvis; these will require your future attention.

Concentrate for the moment with the muscle group that lies parallel to your spinal column. Get acquainted with it. Pincer it and perform push-pulls. Is it stiff and adherent to the spinal column? Perform finger sweeps. Do you find painful, hard, fibrotic thickenings? How about the overlying skin? Is it thick and adherent? Explore the spinal column. Can you feel the contour of each vertebrae, or is the spinal column covered with thick, cartilaginous tissue? This will require extensive treatment to reduce.

Follow your spinal column down to your tailbone. Do you find thick and painful bands of cartilaginous tissue covering the bones of that area? If so, these will require patient, extensive treatment using thumb and finger circles, back-and-forths, and nudges.

Now explore the gluteal tissue. Straighten your hips to put some slack in those tissues. How does the skin feel? Try ripples. Any thick and adherent areas? What about the deeper tissues? Try thumb and multiple-finger circles and probes. Try jiggles and kneadings. Try pincering with back-and-forths. Look for tight, thick, painful bands. In the gluteal region, these can be as thick as your thumb. Be patient and persistent when you self-treat your back. The effort will be worth it.

Body Contouring / Weight Loss

The tissues of the body: skin, fascia, muscles and ligaments, can become progressively thick and fibrotic over the lifetime of an individual--the result of tissue dysfunction. As tissues thicken, their mass increases and they become heavier. I believe this is because they develop a matrix that attracts and absorbs fluid.

When tissues become thick and heavy, they force the *contours* of the body to change. A step on a scale shows the person she is gaining weight, and a look in the mirror reveals that her contours are changing.

When a person experiencing soft tissue dysfunction reaches her 40's, 50's and 60's, she is aware that her neck, shoulders, arms, legs, and abdomen have increased in girth; that she is heavier; and that her body has grown stiff and painful. She has tried all kinds of diets, but no matter how little she eats, she continues to grow heavier and her body contours continue to change. Doctors erroneously inform her that her increasing size and weight gain is caused by an accumulation of "fat" and her pain to some sort of "arthritis."

When I treat someone who is, let's say, in her 50's, I may notice that her legs and knees are thick and heavy. When I observe this, I always make a point to ask: "I bet you think your legs are fat." She answers: "of course they are." I tell her they are not fat, and that I can prove it. I put some lotion on the thickened tissues at both sides of her knees, and guide her fingers to feel how tight, thick, hard and painful the tissues are--definitely not fat. "Oh, my God!, what is that!" is the invariable response. "It's tissue dysfunction," I tell her.

64

So far, over many years, there has not been an exception to the above outcome of this demonstration. I am continually astonished that so many women, and the doctors advising them, confuse the results of soft tissue dysfunction with that of supposed fat.

When I treat someone for chronic pain, I notice that as healing takes place, her contours change. She becomes slimmer, and at last begins to lose those extra pounds. The following case history illustrates this dramatically.

Case History

A woman in her early forties came for treatment because of severe pain throughout her body. She also complained of fatigue and a feeling that her body was getting "tighter." She said she felt her skin was so tight that she was having difficulty moving. She stated that she had to pull herself slowly up stairways by using the stair rails. In addition to all this, she said she was deeply depressed.

When I examined her, I found appreciable thick, contracted, fibrotic tissue throughout her body. She responded well to treatment, and in two weeks her pain was significantly reduced, as was her feeling of fatigue and tightness. However, her depression remained. When we discussed this, she stated that she was depressed because of her "weight problem." She related that when she was married, twenty years earlier, she had a trim figure; her husband could put his hands around her waist, but over the years she had gradually gained too much weight for him to do so.

She said that for the past two years he had not demonstrated romantic interest in her because she had become "so fat." Formerly, men would glance at her figure; now they paid no attention. She had lost her self-image of being an attractive female. Indeed, her body was rotund and pear-shaped.

Frequently, at this stage of treatment, with pain and other symptoms significantly reduced, I would be thinking about discharging her in the near future. However, as I could still feel thick body tissues, particularly at her abdomen, I thought there might be a possibility that if they could be reduced, then perhaps her body contours might also be reduced. I discussed this with her. I told her that I could not offer a guarantee that we would be successful, but that it might be worth a try. She said to go ahead.

65

I continued to treat wherever I felt thick, fibrotic tissues that released hidden pain. And here is when an interesting treatment pattern developed. I would work for forty minutes, then she would excuse herself to go to the lavatory. She returned and stated that she had voided a large amount of urine. Another forty minutes, followed by another large voiding.

This treatment dynamic continued in two hour sessions, three times a week, for the next eight weeks. At the end of this time, to her delight, she once again had a trim figure. She was then discharged from treatment, pain-free, slim, and happy. I chanced to meet her two years later. She still looked trim and stated that she felt very feminine.

The Schatz Technique™ Instructions

Contouring the abdomen: Get lotion and a cup of warm water ready. Start session lying face-up. Apply lotion to the area of your abdomen just below your ribs. Place the palm of your treating hand on your abdomen and use your fingers to explore and normalize thickened tissues (placing your palm on your abdomen prevents fatigue and allows your fingers to be more relaxed, gentle and precise in their movements).

Start with three-finger circles. Then, back and forths. Then side to sides. Take your time, be patient, don't rush. Your fingers are looking for anything that is firm, thick or hard. (Let's turn that around, and say that anything that is not soft or supple should attract your attention--your goal is to get all your tissues to become soft and supple).

Keep in mind that the act of "gently exploring" is the very thing that brings tissues to a healthy condition. Attempting to "force" tissues to become healthy by rubbing or massaging them, does not work. It may require a leap of faith to accept that being gentle can be powerful--however, this is the heart of the Schatz Technique. And, the more you explore and treat, the more effective your gentle explorations will become--experience is the best teacher.

Explore all areas of your abdomen, from the ribs above, to the pelvis, below. Then, turn to one side, and explore and treat, and then to the other side, explore and treat. Every position provides additional treatment opportunities. If your contour change is secondary to tissue dysfunction, you will have undoubtedly found abundant amounts of hidden pain--some

66

may have been surprisingly severe. The more you treat, the less the pain will become, until you are pain-free. As you gain experience, you will find that gentle explorations will discover thickened tissues deep within your body. With gentle persuasion, these will soften and become supple and healthy. Treat your skin with repeated "skin ripplings" (refer to Glossary).

I like to finish each contour session with "planings" (refer to Glossary). Planing is particularly effective in reducing contours. It takes experience to perform it effectively, but you can do it--just be patient. When you get it right, you will find that the skin in the area treated will begin to exfoliate (shed, or flake off) and will do so for a surprisingly long time as you continue the planing. Perform planing on an area in which you have just applied some lotion, and then wiped it off with a towel to get a nice amount of friction. The more experience you have using this technique, the better you will become in performing it.

Contouring the hip, thigh and knee: Perform movements as above. You will find a thickened band of painful tissues running from your hip joint down along the brim of your pelvis. Use three-finger circles and back and forths. Take your time, this area can be stubborn.

Go back to the hip and follow the tissues from the hip, down the outer border of your thigh, to your knee. These tissues are the components of the "knee destroyer" mentioned elsewhere in this book. Thorough treatment of these tissues is extremely important, not only for enhanced body contours, but for maintenance of healthy hip and knee joints. Treat both sides and top and bottom of your thighs and knees. Pay particular attention to the where thigh tissues attach just below your knees. If you suffer chronic knee pain, these tissues probably are the cause.

Contouring the face: perform movements as above, and refer to "treating the face" on page 155. Nothing is so gratifying as having a friend say "my, you are looking so much better--have you lost some weight?"

Breast Pain

Tight, contracted tissue of the breast can cause severe pain. This problem frequently responds quickly to the Schatz Technique.

Case History

A woman in her forties was referred to me for treatment of severe and constant pain of her left breast. She had suffered the agonizing pain for nine years and was convinced that cancer was the only thing that could cause such excruciating pain, although three mammograms were negative. For those nine years, she had been treated by doctors with pain medication and anti-inflammatory medications. But during all those years, her pain had grown increasingly more severe, more unbearable. Finally, a nurse practitioner who knew of my work obtained a referral allowing me to treat.

Examination revealed thick, contracted tissue running from her left pectoral area down into her entire left breast. After a few minutes of treatment, as her tissues softened and her pain eased, she told me that at last she realized that she did not have cancer.

She responded well to treatment and was discharged after four treatments, pain and symptom free.

The Schatz Technique™ **Instructions**

All possibility of underlying organic problems such as cancer must be medically ruled out. Lie with your upper body propped up with pillows or a bolster. Apply lotion up around your collarbone. Treat the skin first, with ripples and thumb sweeps. Let your fingers look for areas of skin that are painful, thick, and adherent to underlying tissues. When found, release them with nudges and gentle single finger probes. Work over the entire breast.

Support the breast upwards with one hand, and with the other make single-finger and multiple-finger sweeps along the bottom of the breast. Pay particular attention to this area, especially if your breast is large and heavy. Use plenty of lotion. The tissues here can become surprisingly thick, hard, and painful.

Go back up to the collarbone area and explore the underlying tissues with multiple-finger circles, back-and-forths, thumb sweeps, and kneadings. You are likely to find excruciatingly painful areas up where your collarbone meets your shoulder joint. Hidden pain can radiate from there *down* into your breast. Work down into the rest of your breast with similar maneuvers. Treat with the breast supported with your other hand, and also with it unsupported, for the greatest variety of treatment effects. Finish each treatment with waves.

Bunions, Plantar Fasciitis, Morton's Neuroma

Medical Approach to Bunions, Plantar Fasciitis and Morton's Neuroma:

Doctors perform surgery on soft tissues and bones of the foot.

Doctors inject drugs into the foot.

Doctors remove or permanently deaden nerves in the foot.

Doctors give names to areas of contracted tissues that press on nerves and cause pain. Bunions, plantar fasciitis and Morton's neuroma are grouped together in this book because the condition (contracted tissues) underlying these three "doctor-names" is confined to the relatively small area of the foot. Treatment technique is the same for all, with variations of emphasis depending on where greater tissue contraction occurs.

Bunions form when tissue contraction pulls the *tip* of the large toe inward, leveraging the *base* of the toe outward, resulting in a painful and unsightly "bump." Plantar fasciitis is caused largely by contracted tissues extending from heel to ball of foot. Morton's neuroma concerns contracted tissues in the ball of the foot. **Its all contracted tissues.**

In order to have a healthy and pain-free foot, all contracted areas have to be normalized. *Surgery, injection of drugs, and removal of nerves do not normalize contracted tissues.*

Case histories for these doctor-names will now be presented, followed by *The Schatz Technique™* treatment instructions.

Case History 1

A woman called and asked if I could help her "bunion problem." She told me she was in her early fifties and that for several years the bunion on her right foot had become increasingly painful. The problem started in a small area that hurt when it rubbed against her shoe.

The pain was now excruciating. She was aware of an ache and tightness when she awoke in the morning, and unbearable pain when she put on a shoe or took a step. Her doctor told her she needed surgery. She declined this and instead had obtained a referral allowing me to treat.

When I examined her, I noted that the contracted tissue of her right foot, caused the tip of her toe to be drawn inward and the base of the toe twisted outward to form a bunion.

The tissues attached to the base of her big "great" toe were thickened and extremely painful to the lightest touch. Severe pain was elicited when I gently attempted to realign the toe. The skin overlying the area was hard and plastic-like and was adherent to underlying tissues.

When I palpated the rest of her foot, I found that all the tissues were tight and thick. I discovered hidden pain areas throughout her foot and up into her calf. She was surprised by all the severe pain she had been unaware of. The tissues of her left foot were also tight and thick, and the big toe was slightly misaligned. She said she was having some pain there, but nothing like the other foot. As we chatted, I learned that she suffered from headaches, sinus pain, tight and painful arms and legs, and her neck and back hurt. Here was another case of global dysfunction.

I spent the two hours of the first treatment on her right foot. I treated the entire foot but concentrated on the skin and underlying tissues surrounding her big toe. By the end of the session, she was able to wear her shoe and bear weight with "very little" pain. She was pleased and encouraged by the results of just one treatment.

When she arrived for her second treatment, she reported that her bunion was much improved. She had not experienced the usual morning ache and tightness, and the pain of walking was less. I again concentrated on the tissues surrounding her right big toe, but spent an increasing amount of time on the rest of her foot. By the end of the treatment, the skin overlying the base of the toe was soft and supple and moved easily over the underlying tissues. I could manually align her toe to a normal position without producing any pain, although it had a tendency to drift back to its old misaligned position.

I suggested that she continue treating her foot between sessions in the manner she had observed so as to speed up recovery. I was able to spend a few minutes on her left foot. Although she was aware of little overt pain, we did find considerable hidden pain.

When she reported for her third treatment a week later, she said that she was extremely pleased with her progress. Her toe remained in proper alignment and she no longer had any pain. I extended treatment to her calves. I continued treatment at decreasing frequency for the next two months. At the end of this time, the tissues of both feet and legs were soft and supple, she had no pain, and her toes were properly aligned.

Case History 2

A woman called and said she was a massage therapist who had terribly painful bunions. She told me her feet were so painful that she could no longer wear regular shoes but had to shuffle around in sandals fitted with thick gel pads. Her podiatrist suggested surgery, which she wanted to avoid, and she asked if I might be able to help her.

I told her I would need a referral from her podiatrist or from her physician in order to examine and treat. She said she would get one and we set up an appointment, two hours on each foot, for the following Monday. She arrived on Monday bearing a referral from her physician--her podiatrist had declined to sign one. She walked slowly and painfully in very wide, flat, loosely strapped gel-padded sandals. She told me that her problem had progressed over the past year and had gotten so bad that even walking in those gel-padded sandals caused excruciating pain. The thought of having surgery on her feet frightened her but she was now seriously considering it.

Something that concerned her almost as much as her painful feet was the fact that she was a Western line-dancer, and for several months had been unable to do any dancing, let alone wear high-heeled boots. Footwear with even a very low heel caused unbearable pain. She feared she would never be able to wear boots again.

72

I examined her feet and noted that each did have a bunion. The tissues of both feet were extremely tender to light touch. I treated each foot for two hours. Her tissues responded well and quickly became soft, pliable with no sign of bunions. When she stepped down from the treatment table and took some steps she was delighted to find that she no longer had any pain. She was able to remove the gel pads and tighten her sandal straps and walk without pain. We scheduled another session for Friday.

When she arrived for her Friday appointment, I was astonished to find her wearing extremely tight, very high-heeled Western boots! She told me her feet had remained free of pain, and felt comfortable in her boots. I treated her and found that her tissues had remained soft and pliable with no return of tightness. I told her there was no need for further treatment, but to call me if there was any return of symptoms.

That was several years ago...no call yet.

Case History 3

I was treating a woman for a bunion on her left foot. Things had gone well, and after a month of treatment she was about to be discharged. She no longer had any pain, the bunion had disappeared, and we were finishing her final treatment. She told me how pleased she was with the condition of her foot.

She also told me that she had an appointment with her podiatrist for a "callous removal." She said removal of the callous, on the skin next to the now disappeared bunion, was an ongoing procedure. Every few months the callous reappeared and had to be removed by her podiatrist. I was aware of the thick callous, however, as the tissues under the callous were now soft and pain-free I hadn't thought much about it. But now I became curious and wondered if I might be able to have an effect on it.

It crossed my mind that the callous had been reforming because the tissues *under it* had been hard and contracted. I wondered if I focused attention on the callous that I could get it softened. I mentioned this to her, and she said to go ahead and try. And, so, for the next forty-five minutes I concentrated on the callous.

At the end of that time, to my surprise, the callous was completely gone-- the skin smooth and soft--no scrapping, sanding or trimming had been necessary. She was now doubly delighted. I told her that I was interested to find if the callous would no longer return, and that I would appreciate it if she might call me in a few months to let me know. She *was* kind enough to call a few months later to inform me that neither the bunion nor the callous had reappeared.

I learned from this experience that callouses are not exclusively caused by skin being rubbed on hard surfaces. Instead, they can be the result of hard, contracted tissues under the skin pushing outward. Now, whenever I see a callous, I consider it a flag of tissue dysfunction deep down.

Plantar Fasciitis
Case History

A gentleman in his forties called. He said that he had suffered severe plantar fasciitis for two years and that his foot pain had progressively worsened. He heard of my work, and asked if I could help him. I told him I would need a referral from a podiatrist or physician in order to examine and treat. He said he would get one, and we set up an appointment for the following Monday.

When he arrived for treatment, I learned that he had already seen a physical therapist who had given him exercises, stretches, and sessions of ultra sound. None of these modalities had helped. He had been given a night splint to stretch the bottom of his foot, but this caused an increase in pain, so he stopped using it. His doctor had given him pain-relievers and an injection of cortisone--no help from these. He had been given an orthotic arch support which helped some when he walked, but his pain and discomfort continued to worsen.

I examined his foot and found that the tissues of his heel were thickened and extremely painful to light touch. Indeed, all the tissues of his foot, from heel, through the arch and into his toes were tight and painful. After two hours of treatment he stated that the pain had lessened, but it still hurt when he put weight on it.

We arranged for two more treatments that week. When he arrived for his second treatment, he said that his pain following the previous treatment was less that evening, but the next morning the pain had returned.

We continued treatment, at decreasing intervals, for the next six weeks. During this time, I explored and found contracted tissues on the top of his foot--extending into his shins. I also found contracted tissues in his Achilles tendon extending into his calf. At the end of the six weeks, all tissues, in his foot, shin and calf had been normalized and were free of pain. He no longer needed the orthotic, and could walk bare-footed on hard surfaces. He was discharged, a very Happy Camper!

Morton's Neuroma
Case History

A woman called and said she was suffering from a Morton's neuroma in her right foot. She had been given a variety of treatments, but the pain had worsened. Her orthopedic doctor said that at this point there were only two treatment options remaining, permanently deaden the nerve in her foot with an injection of chemicals, or remove the nerve with an operation. The choice was hers.

She decided to have the nerve deadened with chemicals, and made an appointment with the doctor to have it done, when a friend told her of my work. She was calling to see if I could offer a less drastic way to go. I told her I would need a doctor's referral in order to examine and treat. She said she would postpone her nerve-deadening procedure and give me a try. And, so, we set up an appointment.

She arrived at the appointed time bearing the necessary referral. Her orthopedic doctor had declined to sign one, but her primary doctor, with some reluctance, had signed the form that allowed me to treat.

I learned that she had been suffering pain in the ball of her foot for three years. At first she only experienced occasional pain. As time went on, the painful episodes had increased in frequency and intensity. Now, she *always* felt a sharp, burning, excruciating pain when she put weight on her foot.

Her orthopedic doctor had injected cortisone into the neuroma. She had been to a physical therapist who had given her stretching exercises and ultrasound treatments. She had been advised to wear a wide shoe and had been given a gel insert to put inside the shoe. She was now using a raised pad to relieve pressure on the neuroma. None of these things had helped, which was why she finally was resigned to have her nerve permanently deadened.

When I examined her foot, I noted a thick, hard, knot in the ball of her foot. This knot (her "Morton's neuroma"), and the area close to it, was tender to light touch. I also noted that the *entire* ball of her foot was stiff, thick and rigid. I was unable move the bones of her feet as they passed through this area. They were locked tightly by rigid tissues.

The tissues of the rest of her foot were surprisingly soft and healthy. This allowed me to focus the entire treatment time on the knot and the rigid tissues of the ball of her foot.

Her tissues responded well, I could feel them rapidly softening. By the end of the two hour treatment, the treated tissues were considerably softer. I could move the bones of her feet--they were no longer held tightly by rigid tissues.

I asked her to step down and see if her foot felt any better. She was surprised and delighted to find that when she put full weight on her foot she felt very little pain. She said there was still some pain, but it was much less. She couldn't believe that there could be so much improvement with just one treatment.

I continued treating twice a week for the next four weeks. By that time the knot had completely disappeared and the tissues surrounding it were soft, supple and free of pain. She no longer had to use a gel insert or raised pad. She was discharged, a very delighted person. She said she was going to call her orthopedic doctor and tell him about my treatment. She was sure he would refer patients to me. However, I never heard from him.

The Schatz Technique™ Instructions

As mentioned in the introduction, what doctors *call* "bunions," "plantar fasciitis" and "Morton's neuroma" are all areas of contracted tissues. These contracted tissues have to be located and normalized so pain will go away and stay away.

Let's assume your right foot is the painful one. Cross your legs so your right foot is resting on your left knee. If you have difficulty doing this because your hip or knee is stiff, you will have to treat those areas first-- refer to those sections of the book for treatment suggestions.

You can start by exploring any part of your foot. Let's begin with the ball of your foot. Have lotion and a cup of water ready.

Rest the outside edge of your <u>right</u> wrist on the inner ankle of your foot--this will put your fingers on the top of your foot and your thumb on the bottom of your foot. Place the palm of your left hand on the outer edge of your foot--this will also put your thumb on the bottom and your fingers on top.

These are good *exploring* positions--and, by placing/resting your hands as suggested, they will be relaxed and won't fatigue easily.

Apply some lotion and use your thumbs to explore the ball of your foot. Have each thumb do separate circles. Then, each thumb do separate up-and-downs (toward toes, then toward heel). Now, bring your thumbs toward each other--attempt to ripple the skin of your ball of foot. If the tissues are stiff/thick/contracted you won't be able to do this at first. Keep at it--your tissues will soften.

Now try wiggling the tissues back and forth by using the fingers of your left hand to press and release the top of your foot toward and away from you--do this several times. Go back to using your thumbs doing circles and up-and-downs. If you have what doctors call Morton's neuroma, use gentle explorations to gently soften it and the tissues around it.

Always be aware of what the tissues under your thumbs and fingers feel like. When you are aware of how tissues *feel*, you are exploring--not rubbing or massaging. Exploring provides just the right amount of pressure that allows tissues to become healthy and painfree again. Be patient--don't rush--your tissues will respond.

Now use your right thumb to gently push and release the base of your big toe forward and backward.

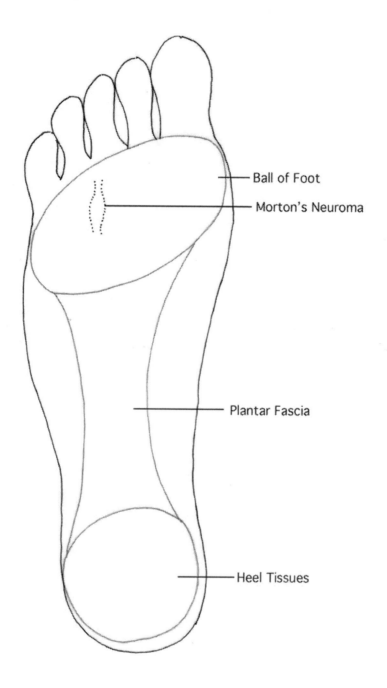

Ball of Foot

Morton's Neuroma

Plantar Fascia

Heel Tissues

Now use both your thumbs to do circles all along your big toe. Do small circles and large circles. If you have a "bunion" pay particular to this area.

Replenish the lotion whenever necessary, or use the drying lotion to provide a bit of friction to your exploring. Also, try dipping your fingers into the cup of water and applying a few drops to see how that feels.

(By the way, if all this is sounding complicated, don't worry--its really very simple--its just applying lotion and exploring with different movements. The more you do, the better you will become.)

Now move your thumbs back toward your heel, exploring as you go. Use your thumbs to make long sweeps back and forth, from ball of foot back to heel. Then small circles, with the tips of your thumbs pointing toward each other--from ball of foot to heel. Once again, from ball of foot to heel. Gently repeat this and the other movements. Now focus attention on the heel itself. Use small thumb circles. When you find areas of pain, be even more gentle with your explorations. You are normalizing the tissues of what doctors call plantar fasciitis.

When you are treating your heel, let your fingers follow any contracted/painful tissues they find. If they lead you up your Achilles tendon and up into your calf--treat and normalize those tissues.

Let's not forget the tissues on the *top* of your foot. It is very likely you will find some extremely painful tissues there (you probably were not aware you had pain on the top of your foot until you explored. These are "hidden pain" areas mentioned earlier in the book). Explore and treat these, and let them lead you up into the tissues of your shins. Explore and treat all painful/contracted tissues you find.

Go back and repeat what you have done since you started. The more you explore and treat the healthier and less painful your feet will become--until all pain is gone and your feet feel great.

An important word of caution! Whenever treating your leg, particularly your calf, check first to see if it seems unusually warm, red or swollen. If so, do not treat and see you doctor immediately. This could be a sign of a serious health condition know as DVT (deep vein thrombosis) that could be life-threatening. Indeed, even if these warning signs are absent, I strongly suggest that readers visit their doctors before treating their legs to rule out any possibility of having this condition.

Bursitis

The term "bursitis" is vague and misleading. It is commonly misused by doctors as a diagnosis of convenience, much as the diagnosis of arthritis is frequently misused. The purpose is to put a name, any name, on an area of pain in order to imply knowledge, when knowledge is absent.

Some joints of the body are contained within a sac. Frequently, when someone complains of pain perceived to be coming from a joint, this sac, or bursa, is blamed as the culprit. This is rarely the case. The cause of pain is usually tight, contracted body tissues *outside* the joint.

Case History

A gentleman in his early sixties was referred to me with a diagnosis of "bursitis of the right hip." He had developed pain in a small area of his hip over a six-month period which had progressively worsened, and it was now severe and constant. He received anti-inflammatory medication and an injection of cortisone, without any reduction of symptoms.

When I palpated the tissues of his hip and thigh, I found tight, contracted, fibrotic tissues from his hip down to his knee. I worked on those tight tissues for two hours. When the gentleman got up and walked about, he no longer experienced any pain.

When he returned for further treatment two days later, some pain had returned, although not to the level of the first treatment. I continued to treat twice a week for six weeks. At the end of that time, the contracted tissue throughout the treated area was softened and supple, and he was discharged, pain and symptom free.

What had been diagnosed as bursitis was a symptom of pain perceived at his hip but caused by contracted tissue throughout his lower extremity.

The Schatz Technique™ Instructions

Soft tissue dysfunction causing the misdiagnosis of bursitis can occur at areas throughout the body. Joints frequently misdiagnosed as having bursitis are those of the shoulder, hip, and knee. Refer to "Carpal Tunnel Syndrome," "Hip Pain and Degenerative Joint Disease," and "Knee Pain" for Schatz Technique treatment.

Cancer While I do not treat cancer, ... a possible pain and cancer connection.

Soft tissue dysfunction frequently underlies chronic pain. Of course, there are other causes of pain, such as cancer. However, pain generated by soft tissue dysfunction may coexist with organic pain, and may even be the primary pain contributor. Patients may suffer needlessly because the soft tissue component of their pain is not addressed. **While I do not treat cancer, the following case provides an interesting look at a possible pain and cancer connection.**

Case History

I was successfully treating a woman for a shoulder problem, and she was pleased with her rapid progress. At her second treatment, she said that since I had been so successful in treating her painful shoulder, could I help her sister-in-law?

She went on to tell me that her sister-in-law was suffering from advanced bone cancer. She had just returned home from a hospital, and was being cared for by a hospice group. The bone cancer had advanced to such a point that her sister-in-law was suffering continuous, excruciating pain in her lower back, which increased significantly with the slightest movement. The pain was uncontrolled by medication except at levels that caused her to become lethargic and unresponsive. Not only was her sister-in-law suffering, but her pain was causing anguish for her husband and other loved ones. My patient asked if I could help.

I said, no, I couldn't help cancer pain, that I treated soft tissue dysfunction and pain associated with soft tissue dysfunction. Pain caused by bone cancer was something I couldn't help. But she persisted, saying they had tried everything else, and her sister-in-law was still suffering. They couldn't turn her in bed without her crying out in pain, and could I please go and see if there was anything I could do to ease her pain. Reluctantly, I told her I would call the hospice group, and see if they would get me a doctor's order to treat, but I was doubtful I could do anything.

The hospice group got the order for me, and that evening I went, although with great trepidation. I took a microcurrent unit, thinking this electronic device was the only thing that might have a chance of easing the woman's pain. I found the sister-in-law lying in bed on her back, grim-faced with pain. Her family was gathered around her. I told them the unit I had brought with me *might* be able to help.

I carefully reached under her to place the electrodes. To my surprise, I found tight, contracted, and fibrotic tissue in her low back. As I gently touched the area, I asked if that was where she was hurting. She said yes.

Instead of using the microcurrent, I applied some lotion and proceeded to gently work on the contracted tissue. After forty minutes, I felt the tissues soften, and I asked if she could move. To her surprise and joy, she moved easily with very slight discomfort. She was able to sit up without pain. She and her family were delighted.

I told them I would not be able to come back on a regular basis and that it was likely the area would tighten again, at least to some extent. I reassured them that I would show the hospice group what I had done so they could continue the treatment if necessary.

The next day, I called the hospice group and told them what I had done and that I would be glad to demonstrate the treatment. The nurse on the phone sounded skeptical that I had been able to help a "bone-cancer pain" with "massage." At the very least, she was not interested enough to take me up on my offer to show her and the other nurses what I had done. I had discharged my patient after her second visit and didn't hear again from her, her sister-in-law, or the hospice group.

The doctors and nurses had confused the severe pain caused by contracted soft tissue squeezing pain receptors with the *assumption* the pain was caused by the bone cancer.

If a doctor happens to read this, perhaps now he will realize why some patients complain of pain so severe they think they have cancer, and yet nothing shows up on their X-ray or other tests. If the doctor carefully touches the tissues of these patients, he will begin to understand why they are hurting so much.

I have had little experience in treating individuals who have cancer, and those were in a rehabilitation setting, not for the treatment of pain they might have been experiencing. The above case history is the one exception. It may well be that pain of soft tissue origin is confused with the pain caused by cancer in other individuals. Refer to the section that corresponds to where your pain is occurring and see if you find tissue dysfunction there that lessens when you apply *The Schatz Technique*™. But before you treat, discuss this with your oncologist; there may be medical reasons that *The Schatz Technique*™ should not be performed.

If, for any reason, you choose not to perform *The Schatz Technique*™ with the intent of reversing dysfunction, gentle sweeps and floats will provide a gentle, soothing effect. This might be an occasion for you to relax and let a friend or loved one apply warm lotion with a loving touch.

"Carpal Tunnel Syndrome"

We are told that carpal tunnel syndrome, the terror of computer operators and many others, is caused by repetitive motion of the wrist and that the best "treatment" for carpal tunnel syndrome is the use of wrist splints, rest, exercise, and the injection of cortisone into the wrist. If these procedures fail, surgery will be necessary, and if one surgery is not successful, then additional surgeries will have to be performed. If carpal tunnel syndrome has become too severe, the condition is irreversible; even surgery cannot help. (If you doubt the accuracy of these statements, ask any doctor.)

False Notions about "Carpal Tunnel Syndrome"

The above statements reflect false notions doctors have about what they call carpal tunnel syndrome. Doctors produce a "diagnosis" of carpal tunnel syndrome by provocative testing of the median nerve *at the wrist* as a way to "prove" dysfunction *at the carpal tunnel*. (Note to reader: the carpal tunnel is not located at the wrist. It is approximately one inch beyond the wrist, at the palm of the hand).

Provocative testing is when doctors brusquely bend their patients' wrists up and down into harsh angles and vigorously press, prod, and tap their patients' median nerves at their wrists. If a patient has the misfortune to experience pain or numbness from the doctor's actions, the doctor concludes there is a problem in the carpal tunnel (again, which is located at the palm) and that surgery will likely be required.

Restricting one's attention exclusively to a tiny bit of tissue that lies beyond the wrist does not make medical sense. Doctors do not carefully examine the soft tissues of their patients or listen to their complaints of pain that conflict with their preconceived notions. They are therefore unaware of what causes their patients' pain.

Think about it. Doctors do not perform this bending, pressing, tapping, and prodding at the actual site of the "tunnel" (on the palm). They "provoke" the median nerve at the wrist *before* it enters the carpal tunnel. They do not know if there is a problem with the carpal tunnel, or, and this is of extreme importance, the precise nature of any problem that may exist. For them, it is all speculation.

Electrophysiological testing is no better. Many individuals who display abnormal electrical findings do not have symptoms, and many others who do have symptoms have perfectly normal electrical findings.

What this means is that doctors have not demonstrated the need for surgery when their patients are rushed to operating rooms to have sharp scalpels slice into their carpal tunnels. Surgery performed without diagnostic justification is surgical mutilation. I consider it a form of malpractice.

If It's Not Carpal Tunnel Syndrome, What Is It?

Restricting one's attention exclusively to a tiny bit of tissue that lies beyond the wrist does not make medical sense. As mentioned throughout this book, doctors do not carefully examine the soft tissues of their patients or listen to their complaints of pain that conflict with their preconceived notions. They are therefore unaware of what causes their patients' pain.

With very few exceptions, such as rare bony abnormalities, fractures, or temporary hormonal changes that occur during pregnancy, extensive soft tissue dysfunction is the cause of the pain. The use of lotion as a discovering or connecting agent is of vital importance to carefully examine the body tissues of the pain sufferer. When this is done, tissue dysfunction will be found throughout the entire upper extremity, from the shoulder down the arm to the elbow, wrist, and hand. The tissues of the neck, back, and chest are also very likely to be dysfunctional. Tissue dysfunction may indeed occur at the carpal tunnel, but this is merely one small part of an extensive problem. The misleading term of Carpal Tunnel Syndrome (CTS) should be replaced with the more accurate and honest one of Extensive Soft Tissue Dysfunction (**ESTD**).

How Does ESTD Develop?

We are told that repetitive wrist movement when we use our computer keyboard is the cause of our problems. That is why doctors prescribe wrist splints--to prevent our wrists from moving. However, if you look down when you are working at your keyboard, you will see that your wrists are **not** moving. It is your fingers that move repetitively. Indeed, it isn't possible to move your wrists at the same time that you type. (Try it.)

Your fingers move repetitively because the muscles connected to them are constantly contracting. These muscles are forced to contract rapidly; 150 times a minute is a conservative estimate. I calculate that at this rate these muscles contract 9,000 times in one hour and 72,000 times in an eight-hour workday. This means that in a five-day week they contract 360,000 times, and in one month, **the muscles contract** 7,200,000 times.

It so happens that these overworked muscles are attached at the elbow. This is where the soft tissue dysfunction starts: *at the elbow.*

As these overworked muscles become increasingly unhealthy, they trigger other muscle groups to become unhealthy. Other tissue systems such as fascia and ligaments are also triggered to become unhealthy. Even the skin throughout the affected area is stimulated to become unhealthy. The problem in terms of tissue systems and areas of the body involved is truly an extensive one.

Nor does this happen overnight. It takes place gradually over a period of weeks, months, and years. It develops so gradually that our bodies are able to accommodate to the significant changes that take place. We are aware of aches and pains and stiffness here and there. At times we may complain of a stiff neck or a sore shoulder or a painful forearm, but a visit to the doctor for pain-killers takes the edge off the pain, thus enabling our pain-sensing center to further adjust to the continuing tissue changes.

One of the many tissues that have been stimulated to become unhealthy is the carpal ligament, the roof of the carpal tunnel. It thickens and contracts and draws the carpal bones closer together, narrowing the cross section of the carpal tunnel, thereby increasing the hydrostatic pressure on the median nerve.

As time goes on and it becomes increasingly thick, it presses down *directly* on the nerve, which lies immediately below, stressing it more and more. The ligament, and the fascia and skin overlying it, eventually become a thickened, hardened, adherent mass that causes even greater stress on the median nerve. As the median nerve becomes progressively stressed, pain, numbness and tingling become more severe.

Because doctors do not know how to properly examine their patients, they do not understand this. They fancy that tendons passing deep in the tunnel somehow swell and press the median nerve up into what they regard as a healthy carpal ligament. In order to relieve the pressure, they sever the ligament.

Bizarre, isn't it? The "gold standard" of medical care that doctors offer patients suffering from what they call carpal tunnel syndrome is to mutilate perceived healthy tissue. Some local relief of pain and other symptoms may result from surgically relieving pressure on the median nerve. However, surgical intrusion may cause nerve damage and bowing of flexor tendons, and post surgical scarring always worsens a soft tissue problem.

Patients with the best of results are very likely to find that their fingers, hands, and arms do not have the strength or agility to return to their original occupation. Indeed, there are those, doctors tell us, whose damage from repetitive motion disorder is so severe that they are permanently disabled and will have to live the rest of their lives in pain, unable to use their hands for any gainful employment. These poor results and gloomy prognoses spring from a lack of knowledge of soft tissue dysfunction. Ignorance leads to improper treatment.

The proper treatment for this extensive problem is to normalize all the dysfunctioning tissue wherever it occurs: neck, back, shoulder, arm, forearm, hand, fingers, thumb. When this is done, the individual becomes pain-free and healthy again and can return to full-time occupation.

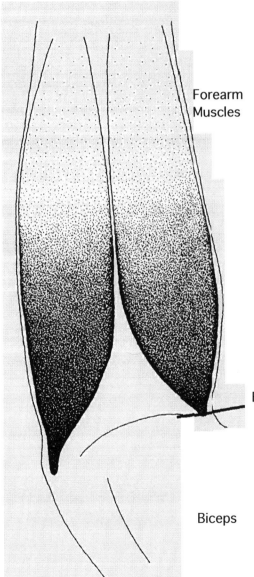

Forearm
Muscles

Elbow

Biceps

If the occupation happens to be particularly stressful, repeat treatments can be given from time to time so the individual can remain healthy and pain-free, can continue to feel great, and can continue to perform his or her job of choice.

The term "Carpal Tunnel Syndrome" is inappropriate and misleading. Extensive Soft Tissue Dysfunction (ESTD) is more accurate and honest. The problem starts when the muscles that move the fingers are overworked. These muscles are located at the elbow. When they become dysfunctional, they send distress signals up and down the arm, triggering other areas to become unhealthy.

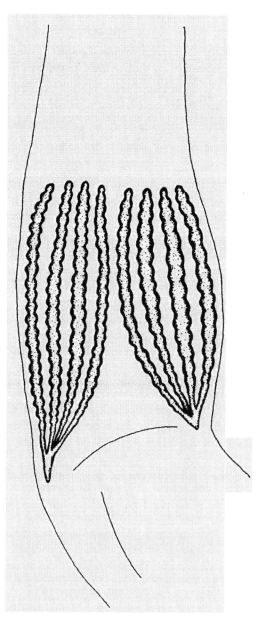

Stressed tissues at the elbow become tight, contracted, and fibrotic.

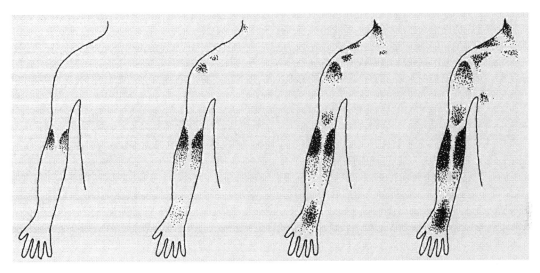

The problem that started at the elbow triggers progressive dysfunction up and down the arm.

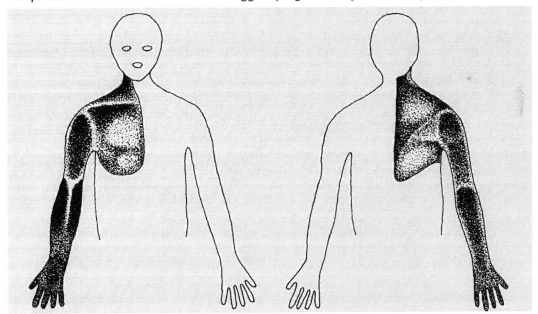

This drawing depicts fully developed ESTD.The problem that started at the elbow now extends up to the neck, back, and chest, and down to the hand.The tissues of the carpal tunnel may be affected, but they are one small area of an extensive problem. All areas must be treated if the individual is to become pain-free and healthy again. Surgery for this soft tissue problem, or any soft tissue problem, is inappropriate. It introduces scarring and may damage nerves and vessels. Surgery does not soften tight, contracted tissues.

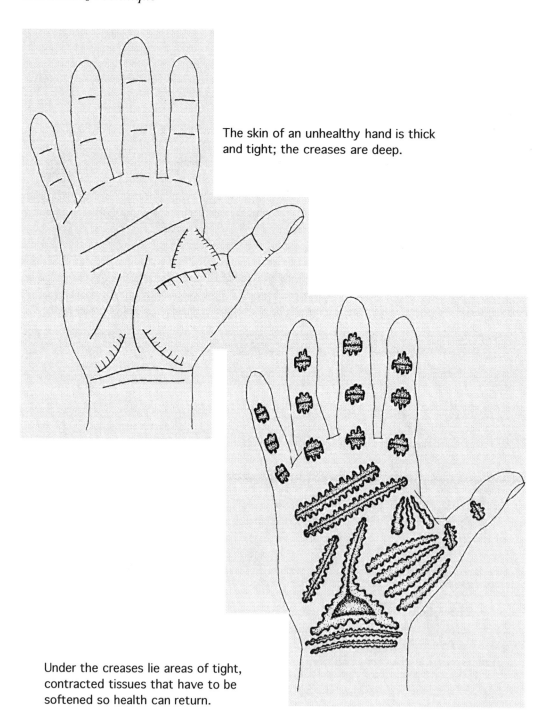

The skin of an unhealthy hand is thick and tight; the creases are deep.

Under the creases lie areas of tight, contracted tissues that have to be softened so health can return.

92

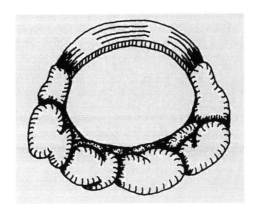

The famous carpal tunnel

Components of the carpal tunnel

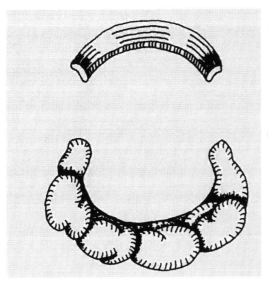

Carpal ligament
(roof of tunnel)

Carpal bones
(sides and bottom)

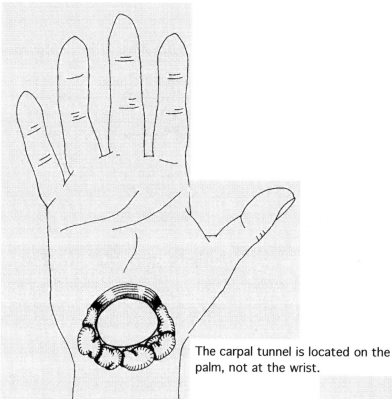

The carpal tunnel is located on the palm, not at the wrist.

Cross sections of the carpal tunnel (not to scale)

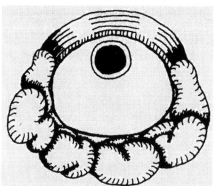

The important median nerve passes through the tunnel immediately below the carpal ligament. For clarity, the tendons that lie deep in the tunnel have been omitted.

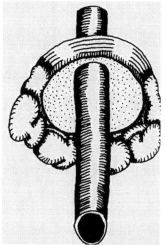

Perspective view of the median nerve passing directly under the carpal ligament

94

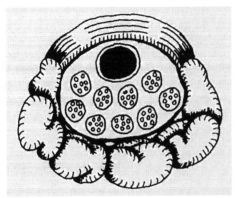

Cross section of the carpal tunnel showing median nerve and the tendons that move the fingers. The median nerve passes directly under the carpal ligament. Finger tendons lie deep in the tunnel.

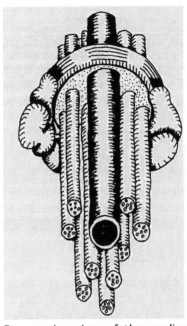

Perspective view of the median nerve and finger tendons as they pass under the carpal ligament.

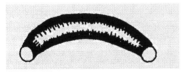

When stimulated by unhealthy forearm tissues, the carpal ligament thickens and contracts.

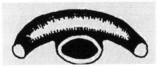

It presses down on the median nerve, squeezing and stressing it.

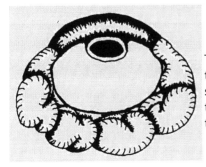

The contracting carpal ligament pulls on the carpal bones, narrowing the cross section of the tunnel. This increases the hydrostatic pressure and stress on the median nerve.

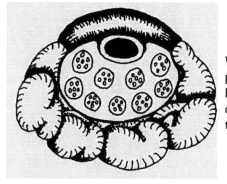

While all of this is happening, the tendons stay in place deep in the tunnel. The median nerve has been stressed by the thickened and contracted carpal ligament (that was triggered by forearm tissues), not by the deep tendons.

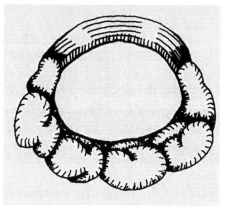

With effective (nonsurgical) treatment, the carpal ligament and all dysfunctioning tissues of the hand, arm, neck, back, and chest become soft, supple, and healthy again.

The Schatz Technique™ **Brand Pain Prevention *and* Treatment Method –An Overview**

Let us say that someone comes for treatment bearing the diagnosis of carpal tunnel syndrome. This is how I treat. I may start my exploration of the patient's tissues at the shoulder and work down the arm. Or, I may start at the hand and explore upward. For this example I will start at the shoulder. Lotion is applied, and I feel for tight, contracted tissue. I work gently. One can work gently but still move tissues deep in the body. When tight tissues are found, they are coaxed to relax, to let go.

A process of the patient getting acquainted with his or her body begins. The gentle touch awakens pain that has lain dormant for perhaps years. A variety of techniques–all gentle, all involving exploring and coaxing is used. As the awakened pain subsides, healing has begun.

Treatment continues down the arm. The patient is usually surprised at the large amount of pain that has been stored up at the elbow. I work very gently there. The forearm reveals severely thickened and painful tissue. I work thoroughly there. Before I get to the wrist, patients frequently tell me that the pain and tingling in their hand and fingers have subsided significantly, or has gone away entirely. This surprises them greatly.

We are now at the hand. The hand is the end point, the downstream terminus of all the complex of dysfunction that lies above it. The skin of a dysfunctioning hand is thickened and tight. The joints of the palm, fingers, and thumb are bound down by thick tissue that has a hard scar like consistency. The creases of the joints are deep, thick, and painful to light touch. The tissue just beyond the wrist, at the base of the palm, is severely thickened and feels like a piece of rigid plastic. The skin is adherent to this hard, thick area. When gently pressed, the patient frequently feels increased pain and tingling of the thumb and first two fingers.

This is the area of the carpal tunnel. Instead of mutilating it with a sharp knife as a doctor would do, with *The Schatz Technique*™ it is gently kneaded and coaxed to relax, to soften, to become *healthy* again. We move on to the palm proper, and the thumb and fingers.

It is surprising how frequently, even at the very first treatment, that the patient feels a significant response to this gentle work. I have had patients tell me their pain has gone down seventy-five percent by the end of their first treatment. Some no longer have any pain and their entire arm feels lighter and more alive. Not only that, their fingers are less stiff and move in a more normal manner.

The moments have flown by. We have made a good start. At the next visit, we will do more. We will treat the same areas, but, as they have already begun to soften and normalize, we won't have to spend as much time on them, so we can move on to the neck and back and perhaps the other arm. Wherever we find tight, contracted tissue, there is where we will treat.

Frequency of treatment depends on the severity of the problem and the patient's response to treatment. I might suggest two to three treatments the first week, reducing as soon as possible to once a week, then perhaps once every two weeks, and so on. I might want to do a recheck in three or four months to make sure there has been no return of tightness. When the patient is finally discharged, all treated areas are soft, supple, pain-free and healthy. The (former) patient now feels great! It is surprising how wonderful a person feels when his body has been properly treated.

Case History 1

Nine years ago, my wife told me that her hairstylist, Theresa, had developed severely painful arms and hands and was no longer able to work. Theresa had an appointment with the hand clinic of a particular teaching hospital the following Thursday. Theresa, I was told, was distraught by all the pain she was having and was fearful and apprehensive about her future. My wife told Theresa that I treated people with severe pain and was apparently successful because so many people called to thank me for helping them. She suggested that Theresa call me, as I might have some suggestions for her.

When I talked with her, she sobbed continuously and there was panic in her voice. She told me that her problem had developed over a two-year period and particularly involved her dominant left arm and hand. The pain had gotten so bad that she could barely lift her arm and could no longer hold a pair of scissors or a blow dryer. In addition, the constant pain was affecting her emotionally. She asked if I could tell her anything that might be of help.

I told Theresa exactly what would happen when she went to the hand clinic. The doctors would put her through all kinds of tests and examinations. Some would be uncomfortable; some would likely be excruciatingly painful. The tests and examinations would probably drag on for two or three weeks and in the end the doctors would not be able to offer her anything that would help her become healthy and pain-free again.

I told Theresa that there was a chance I might be able to help and enable her to avoid the painful and ultimately unproductive tests she would be put through at the hand clinic. I suggested that I treat her on the following Monday, Tuesday, and Wednesday. We would have three days to see if my treatments would be of significant help. If they were, then she would not have to go through the painful procedures at the hand clinic. If my treatments were not successful, then at least my findings might provide information that would help the doctors.

I would need a doctor's referral that allowed me to examine and treat her. I suggested that she call the doctors at the hand clinic, tell them about our conversation, and ask them if they could give her a check-over the following day in order to provide me with a referral to treat. It was my feeling that the doctors at the hand clinic would not give Theresa the referral. It was my experience and observation that doctors did not want to lose control of a patient or a prospective patient, but maybe I would be proven wrong. My schedule was full for the following week, but I knew my patients would be pleased that someone else would have a chance to become pain-free and would not mind being rescheduled.

Theresa said that what I told her made sense and that she would call the doctors. Her voice sounded relieved. We made arrangements to meet at my office on Monday morning at nine.

I arrived at my office early on Monday to set things up. At 8:45 a.m., the phone rang. It was Theresa. She had called the doctors at the hand clinic, and they told her that it is was of extreme importance that she keep her appointment with them on Thursday, as only they had the knowledge and expertise to evaluate her problem and that under no circumstance should she do anything before they told her that she could do it. Theresa apologized for the trouble she had caused with the rescheduling of my patients. She thanked me for my time and trouble. I wished her luck, and we hung up. I felt miffed, largely because I thought I could have helped her and saved her a lot of grief.

Two weeks later, the phone rang. It was Theresa. She sounded even more distraught than before. In between her sobs, she told me that things had gone along exactly as I told her they would. The tests and exams made her pain completely unbearable. Especially horrible were the sharp needles they inserted into her already painful forearms. She told me the doctors had done all the testing but she would have to wait a week for the final consultation, when the chief doctor would tell her about their findings and conclusions and the treatments they would suggest.

Her arm and hand had become so unbearably painful that she couldn't wait the week until the final consultation. She asked if I might be able to schedule her in for anything that might reduce her pain. I reminded Theresa that I needed a referral that would allow me to treat her. She felt confident that the doctors at the hand clinic would understand that she was hurting so badly and would gladly give her a referral for something that might help her pain.

The next morning, I arrived at my office well before the 9:00 A.M. time we had arranged. At 8:45 the phone rang. This time it was Theresa's husband. He told me that Theresa had called the hand clinic, but they told her absolutely not to see anybody or do anything until the final consultation the following week, no matter how "uncomfortable" she was. Theresa's husband apologized. He said he knew this was the second time she had canceled. As a matter of fact, she was too embarrassed to call herself. I told Theresa's husband not to worry. I was deeply sorry she was having so much pain and wished them both luck.

A week later, the phone rang, and it was Theresa again. She said, "Bernard, you won't believe what happened at the final consultation yesterday!" She had asked her husband to accompany her to the final consultation, as she was too nervous and upset to go alone. When they were ushered into the chief doctor's office, he was seated behind his desk, attired in his white jacket, thumbing through her examination and test folder. There was a moment of silence as he finished his perusal of her reports. He then said that he was sorry and saddened to report to them that her case of carpal tunnel syndrome was so severe, that the condition of her hands and fingers was so terrible, that even surgery would not be able to help her. Her case was beyond help.

He *could* tell her that she would have to change careers. She would have to find some line of work in which she wouldn't have to use her hands. He was sorry, but there was nothing that could be done for her. Theresa then asked if the physical therapist for whom she had been requesting referrals might be able to help her.

"Well, yes," replied the doctor, "you might try him."

At this point, her husband got up and approached the doctor. Theresa said that her husband is a mild person but he was so angry she thought he was going to punch the doctor. "You mean to tell us that after all this time, there is nothing you can do? But that maybe the person you had us cancel twice, and probably won't even want to speak to us, might be of some help?" The doctor hurriedly (at last) wrote out the referral, and they left. Her husband did not strike the doctor.

When Theresa came for her first treatment, her face was drawn with pain. She moved her arms and hands guardedly and held the fingers of her hands open and outstretched. She talked slowly and seemed on the verge of tears. She told me her experience at the hand clinic had been a terrible one and that she was deeply depressed and worried about what they had told her. She had been a hairstylist for nineteen years and it was a career she loved. It was the only thing she knew how to do or wanted to do.

After the final consultation at the hand clinic, she and her husband had discussed alternative careers in which she wouldn't have to use her hands. The only thing they could think of was some sort of day care for children. But even with something like that she would have to pick up a child, which presently she was unable to do.

I found that the tissues of her upper and mid-back, her neck, both shoulders, arms, forearms, wrists, hands, and fingers, in addition to the tissues of her left anterior torso, were spasmed, contracted, thickened, fibrotic, and extremely painful to even very mild examination. The tissues of her left upper extremity were more severely affected than her right. The skin overlying these areas was thickened, adherent, and very painful to light touch. She couldn't bend the fingers of her left hand, or hold anything in them. It caused her great pain to drive her car, as she couldn't grip the steering wheel in a normal fashion with either hand.

I treated Theresa for three hours. At the end of this time, she said she felt "great." She was able to bend the fingers of both hands and reported that the pain in her arms and hands was down seventy-five percent. She was extremely pleased with the results of the first visit.

When she came by the next day for her second treatment, she reported that she had been able to drive home after yesterday's treatment with her hands and fingers gripping the steering wheel of her car in a completely normal fashion, without pain.

It is sad that the medical community has so little understanding of the underlying cause of body dysfunction that the neurologists, orthopedic surgeons, and rehabilitation specialists of a prestigious medical teaching hospital doomed Theresa to a life of progressive, crippling pain. Instead, when she received appropriate care, she rapidly became healthy, happy, and pain-free again.

I treated Theresa daily the first week in three-hour sessions. During that week, there was some flare-up of pain here and there, but by the end of the week she was feeling no pain, except an occasional twinge.

Although Theresa was feeling well by that time, she was worried about her return to work the following week. She had not been able to work at all for several days. Her workdays for the previous two or three months had been nightmarish with pain. However, when she came by for treatment following her first day of return to work, she reported that she had been able to perform her regular duties all day without pain, except for a little twinge in her left palm.

I continued to treat Theresa for the next four months at rapidly decreasing treatment frequency.

There were times when she had minor flare-ups of pain, but for the most part, the treatments were directed toward reducing areas of remaining contracted tissue so they would not retrigger pain in the future.

When we discontinued treatment at the end of the four months, Theresa was completely pain-free and feeling very well. Her tissues were soft, supple, and she no longer felt emotionally stressed. She had begun to lift weights again, and she was able to continue her career as a hairstylist.

It is sad that the medical community has so little understanding of the underlying cause of body dysfunction that the neurologists, orthopedic surgeons, and rehabilitation specialists of a prestigious medical teaching hospital doomed Theresa to a life of progressive, crippling pain. Instead, when she received appropriate care, she rapidly became healthy, happy, and pain-free again.

I sent regular reports about Theresa's recovery to her doctor, the one who had told her there was nothing that could be done, that she would have to change careers, and would have to live the rest of her life in pain. However, he did not have the professional interest to ask me to show him what I had done to help her so he could use the information to help his other patients.

Although it has been nine years since I treated Theresa, she remains pain-free, and active in her career as a hairstylist.

Case History 2

An article in a local paper described the plight of a young woman who had severe carpal tunnel syndrome of both wrists. Her condition was so painful and critical that surgery was scheduled for both wrists in two weeks. The article pointed out that she had no medical insurance and was in the process of selling her small business to pay for the surgery.

I phoned her and asked if she would be interested in trying a non-surgical treatment for her carpal tunnel problem. I told her there would be no charge, but I would need a doctor's referral allowing me to treat her. She said she was very interested and that there would be no problem in getting the doctor's referral. She had a wonderful doctor who would be willing to try anything that might help her.

She arrived at the appointed time bearing the referral. She informed me that her doctor wanted to speak with me before I started any treatment. I immediately called him. He told me that under no circumstance was I to do anything that would interfere with the surgery that was scheduled for his patient. I assured him that I understood what he was saying. He said that I could then go ahead and treat her.

The first thing I noticed was her wrist splints. They were filthy. She had been wearing them for several months (if worn continuously for more than a week or two, splints can cause serious immobilization problems). Her doctor had told her to wear one on each wrist at all times. I learned that her fingers, hands, and forearms caused her continual and severe pain and tingling, and that any movement increased the pain to an even higher level. Her hands had grown weak, and she had difficulty doing the simplest task. Driving was dangerous because the pain, weakness, and the cumbersome splints made gripping the steering wheel difficult.

I removed the splints and noted that her fingers, hands, wrists, and forearms were swollen and painful to the lightest touch. The joints of her fingers and palms were thickened, and it was difficult and painful for her to move them even slightly. Her right hand was more painful than her left.

I treated her three times the first week in three-hour sessions. At the end of the first session, she stated that there was less pain and tingling in both hands and wrists, and she could move her fingers more easily.

When she came in for her second session, she was not wearing her wrist splints. Her hands and arms were so comfortable that she felt she didn't need them, she said. She reported that she was able to grip the steering wheel of her car in a "near-normal" fashion. At the end of the second session, she stated that there was no longer any pain or tingling in her left wrist and hand, and only a small amount of pain in her right forearm, and the only tingling was in her right forefinger.

When she came in for her third session, she reported that she was "feeling a lot better all around" and had even felt well enough to resume horseback riding after the previous session, and she had canceled her surgery. She stated that there was "barely noticeable" pain in her right forearm, and a "slight tingling" in the last two joints of her right forefinger. At the end of the third session, she stated that she no longer had any pain or tingling in either hand, wrist, or forearm.

We still had a lot of work to do. Considerable contracted tissue remained, and there was some grip weakness that had to be resolved. I advised her to avoid horseback riding until after discharge, as we didn't want to contend with additional problems that might result from her being thrown from a horse. We agreed to continue our three-times-a-week treatment schedule.

I sent a preliminary report to her doctor describing her improved status, and she went back to him the following week for a recheck. She could hardly wait to show him how improved she was. When she returned for treatment following her doctor's visit, I asked how things went. She told me that she had proudly demonstrated how she could move her hands and arms freely and without pain, and that she had canceled her surgery appointments. I asked what her doctor had said. Her reply: "He didn't say anything."

I continued treating her at decreasing frequency for the next six weeks. She was then discharged, pain and symptom free. I continued reporting to her doctor as treatments continued, but never heard a word from him. I thought he would be interested in finding out what I had done that allowed his patient to avoid those drastic and expensive surgeries he had ordered, but apparently I was wrong.

Case History 3

A young woman stopped by my office. She had recently seen a TV program that had her worried. The program described the symptoms of carpal tunnel syndrome and warned viewers that carpal tunnel syndrome can become *irreversible* if treatment is delayed too long. She told me that she worked for the post office and that her job was to continuously feed envelopes into a mechanical device throughout the workday. Over the past year her hands and arms had become increasingly painful and stiff. Recently the pain had become so severe, and her fingers had become so stiff, that she could no longer ignore the problem. The TV program had convinced her that she had carpal tunnel syndrome and that her condition was now irreversible.

She had an appointment with a doctor who specialized in carpal tunnel syndrome and was going to see him in a few days. In the meantime, someone I had helped suggested she contact me. I told her that I would need a doctor's referral to treat her. She said she would get one the following week from the carpal tunnel syndrome specialist. We arranged for her to see me immediately following her doctor's appointment.

She arrived for her treatment in a state of panic. Her fears had been justified. She did have carpal tunnel syndrome, and it was indeed severe. I noticed that she was wearing a wrist splint on each wrist. The doctor said that, because of the severity of her problem, she was to wear the splints at all times, day and night for the next three weeks. He had written a note to her supervisor, stating that it was important for his patient to completely rest her hands and wrists for three weeks and she was not to report for work during this time. She was to return to him at the end of the three-week period for reassessment. When she asked the doctor for a referral allowing me to treat her, he at first refused, but when she insisted he finally signed one.

She was alarmed, because the doctor said she had waited so long that her carpal tunnel syndrome was now severe. She was concerned about her job because it was a busy season and her supervisor would not be pleased about her absence of three weeks. She dreaded the idea of wearing the uncomfortable wrist splints for three weeks, day and night.

I removed the splints and examined her hands and arms. The tissues of both upper extremities were tight and contracted, but not so much as to incite panic. I had examined and successfully treated tissues that were considerably more dysfunctional than hers. I told her that, although no guarantee could be given, I thought there was a good chance she could achieve a complete recovery.

I worked on her fingers, hands, arms, shoulders, and back for three hours. At the end of this time, the tissues of those areas were appreciably looser and less painful. She was now hopeful that she could be successfully treated. She felt so much better that she thought she didn't need the wrist splints. She asked what I thought. I told her that if the doctor said to wear the splints for three weeks that she had better do so. I added that if it were me that had to wear the splints, I would throw them in the trash can, but she should follow the doctor's orders.

When she returned for her next treatment two days later, she told me that following our first session she had stopped by the doctor's office with the splints he had sold her (she had to pay cash for them) and asked for her money back. There was some reluctance to take back the splints and to return her money, but she had insisted, saying that "because of the good work of Mr. Schatz" she no longer needed them. Finally, her money was returned and the splints were taken back. She continued to do her post office duties and was fairly comfortable even after eight hours of work, and, although she experienced some pain in her hands and arms, "It was nothing like before."

We continued sessions three days a week for the next three weeks. We then reduced their frequency to two days a week for the following three weeks, then down to once a week for a month. Her fingers, hands, and forearms responded well, and rapidly became pain-free. Much of the treatment emphasis was directed toward her upper arms (particularly her right) and her neck. During the entire treatment period, she continued to work full shifts with the mechanical device she had to deal with. At the end of this time, she was discharged from treatment, pain and symptom-free, and feeling great.

She called two months later. She was experiencing some tightness in her shoulders and arms, accompanied by a little pain, and wanted me to work on them before things got worse. I noted some return of tissue tightness and contraction. These responded rapidly and in three two-hour sessions she was once again discharged from treatment.

Another call came six months later. She had worked continuously without pain or discomfort until a few days earlier. The workload with the mechanical device she had to contend with had gotten particularly heavy and there was some return of tightness and some pain in her arms and forearms. Her fingers and hands had continued to do well. A few more treatments and she was pain-free and supple again.

I reported her progress to the doctor–the one that "specialized" in carpal tunnel syndrome–who had reluctantly signed the referral allowing me to treat. I also called him several times, trying to arrange an appointment so I could discuss with him my treatment methods that had nonsurgically reversed and normalized the tissues of someone he had diagnosed as having severe carpal tunnel syndrome. But he never had time to talk with me. Nor did he ever refer a patient for treatment of carpal tunnel syndrome, despite the significant recovery this patient had made without wearing uncomfortable wrist splints or without being subjected to other medical treatments, including surgery, that inevitably follow the diagnosis of "severe carpal tunnel syndrome."

Case History 4

A sixty-two-year-old woman came to me for treatment of her painful hands. A friend had told her of my work, and she had a referral allowing me to treat.

When I took her case history, I learned that carpal tunnel surgery had been performed on both her hands, one surgery on her left hand, and two on her right. Unfortunately, the surgeries had not alleviated the pain of either hand. Her right hand was more painful, which was why the surgeons had tried a second surgery two years prior to her appointment with me.

She told me that in addition to the pain, both her hands had grown increasingly weak. She had difficulty manipulating keys, holding glassware, or using a pen or pencil. Following each surgery, she received physical therapy consisting of warm paraffin dips, stretches, and exercises, but those procedures had not helped her pain or weakness.

She was surprised when I applied lotion to her right shoulder and began exploring the tissues there, because none of the doctors or therapists had touched those tissues. She was further surprised at all the tightness and pain there. I let her feel the lotioned skin of her shoulder, arm, and forearm so she could see how thick the tissues were in those areas and how painful they were to light touch. We found contracted tissues in her hand. The skin was thick and drawn tightly across the palm. The surgical scarring on her palm was adherent to the tissues under it, and her fingers were stiff. I found similar tissue dysfunction on her left side, but not to the same extent.

I treated her daily for two weeks. The first week, I concentrated on her right upper extremity, and the second week on her left side. She responded rapidly to treatment, and at the end of the two-week period she no longer had any pain in either hand, her strength had improved significantly, and she was able to use both hands in a normal manner.

She was delighted with the results and felt she did not need further treatment, although I still felt tight tissues. I told her to call me if any symptoms recurred. No call ever came. I sent a report to the doctor who had signed her referral, describing her dramatic response to my treatments. No call came from him, either.

Why the Silence from the Doctors?

I was invited to speak to an organization of nurses about my approach to the treatment of carpal tunnel syndrome. I had helped the sister of one of their members, which was how they knew of my work. At the meeting, I discussed what I found to be the cause of carpal tunnel syndrome and my approach to treating it. I told them I was surprised I had never received another referral from a doctor to whom I had returned a patient successfully treated for previously untreatable symptoms. Not one doctor had bothered to ask me what I had done to help a patient previously judged to be "unhelpable."

I asked the nurses, all of whom worked closely with doctors, why the doctors never made more referrals? They were unanimous in their response:

• **The doctors did not want to lose control of their patients.**

• **The doctors did not want to admit that they had previously been wrong in their treatment approach.**

• **The doctors did not want to allow someone outside their profession to come up with something better.**

• **The doctors were running a business and didn't want to lose revenue.**

• **The doctors had forgotten why they had become doctors, which was to help people first and foremost.**

The Schatz Technique™ Instructions

I do not know if you have been having problems for an extended time or if your symptoms have surfaced recently. Perhaps you have been subjected to one or more surgeries. Each case has to be treated on an individual basis, so only a generalized approach can be described here.

I am going to assume your problem is with the tissues of your right arm. Your neck, upper back, and chest are probably also involved. Refer to "Migraine and Muscle Contraction Headaches" and "Frozen Shoulder" for *The Schatz Technique*™ suggestions for those areas. *Treatment can start with any involved tissue.* For this example, let's start at your shoulder.

Keep in mind that as your fingers explore and investigate your tissues, they are at the same time treating those tissues. The more your fingers investigate, the more they treat.

You will treat from your shoulder down to your fingertips. Before you start treatment, try this: wiggle the fingers of your affected hand. Wiggle them as fast as you can. It is likely they move slowly, stiffly, and painfully. Now wiggle the fingers of your "better" hand. It is likely these fingers move more freely and wiggle faster than your affected hand. We will recheck these movements following your treatment.

Get into a comfortable sitting position with a towel-covered pillow on your lap and a container of lotion and a cup of warm water next to you. Warm the lotion, if you wish.

Place your forearm and hand on the pillow. This will help to relax the tissues of your upper extremity, making your treatment more effective. Don't hold your elbow away from your body, as this will tense your tissues. Instead, let your arm go slack against your body; this will greatly assist you in your examination and treatment. Keep in mind that as your fingers explore and investigate your tissues, they are at the same time treating those tissues. The more your fingers investigate, the more they treat. Be very gentle, don't try to force anything.

With your left hand, apply a liberal amount of lotion to your shoulder. Use finger and thumb sweeps over your entire shoulder muscle (the deltoid), then doubled-finger circles, and nudges. Let your fingers get acquainted with the tissues there. Are they hard and stringy? Do you find pain there? Adjust the amount of lotion by wiping with a towel, so your

110

sweeps, circles, and nudges have more grip, enabling you to sense the underlying tissues a bit differently. You want to get as much information about those tissues as possible. Explore the muscle, top to bottom, side to side. Move slowly, don't rush.

Pincer the deltoid up at its very top between your thumb and forefinger. Rock it with push-pulls. Go down its entirety to where it attaches, about halfway down your arm, then back up and proceed downward with thumb kneadings. Continue with this up-to-down pattern. Follow the bands of tissues that you feel inside, that run down the length of the muscle. Keep looking for tight and painful areas. This is your first session; you will be busy with all sorts of discoveries as you proceed.

Turn your attention to the skin overlying your deltoid. Explore with skin ripples. Can you find thickened areas of skin? Painful areas? Now try skin graspings. Do you find areas adherent to underlying tissues? Any painful areas? Carefully check the area where the deltoid attaches; you are apt to find thickened, dysfunctioning skin there.

Finish investigation and treatment of your deltoid tissues with overall kneadings. I wager your deltoid is now considerably looser and more supple.

Move down to your biceps tissues. Let's start with the skin. Apply lotion. Grasp the muscle with your fingers on the outside, and your thumb on the inside, up into your armpit. Sweep with thumb to the fingers. Look for thick, crinkly skin; these are signs of skin dysfunction. Remember, wherever you find areas of skin dysfunction, you will invariably find tissue problems underneath that need treatment, so always examine the skin carefully. Do you find painful areas, or areas that become painful after gentle exploration? Use skin graspings, circles, and floats.

When you have examined your skin to your satisfaction, turn your attention to the deeper tissues. Thumb side-to-sides will be useful on the inside tissues that run down from your armpit to the lower attachment of the muscle just beyond the elbow. Use your fingers for back-and-forths on the outside tissues. It is likely that you will find hard, painful, wirelike bands that need softening and normalizing, particularly toward the lower attachment of the muscle. Use single- and multiple-finger circles. Follow with thumb circles. Pincer the muscle and perform push-pulls. Finish with a good overall kneading.

You are ready to turn your attention to the tissues on the opposite side of the biceps; these are the tissues associated with the triceps muscle (the biceps bends your elbow; the triceps straightens it). Start again with skin exploration using skin ripples and graspings. It is likely you will find considerable crinkly skin overlying the triceps. Explore the deeper tissues with nudges, waves, and circles.

It is possible that in your treatment so far, you found areas that triggered sensations down into your hand and fingers, such as increased pain, tingling, or numbness. As you proceed, these hand and finger sensations will undoubtedly increase dramatically because you are now ready to explore and treat the tissues that are primarily responsible for the problems commonly called carpal tunnel syndrome.

You are now going to "work on" (explore) your forearm. The forearm muscles and associated tissues are attached close to the elbow. They move your thumb and fingers, and are the tissues that get overworked. Be prepared to find considerable amounts of overt and hidden pain in these tissues. Remember to always be kind and gentle to your tissues as you explore.

Apply some lotion to the muscle bulge that lies on the thumb side of your forearm. These muscles straighten your fingers and thumb. Work the skin overlying these tissues; thumb sweeps are good. Treat the skin thoroughly, from above the elbow, down to the wrist. Then turn your attention to the tissues underneath. Start with pincering the muscle bulge and gently rock with push-pulls. Follow the bulge from where it starts above the elbow down to where it separates into the various thumb and finger tendons. Then try thumb and finger circles, back-and-forths, and nudges. Learn to trust your fingers; let them suggest what patterns you should use. Look for painful, contracted muscle bands that lead downward. Track these with back-and-forths.

You will likely find a particularly hard, painful band that starts just above the bump at your elbow joint and passes down into your hand next to the bump at your wrist joint.

Most likely, you will find extensive tight, contracted, and extremely painful tissues on this side of your forearm. Are you surprised at what you have found so far? And you haven't even gotten to your hand yet!

You are now ready to explore and treat the other forearm bulge. This contains the muscles that bend your thumb and fingers. Additional surprises await you here. Apply lotion, and be particularly gentle, because these tissues are likely to be more tender than those of the finger straighteners. When you explore these tissues, are you aware of sensations that shoot up your arm, and down into your hand? By the way, how is your hand feeling? Chances are your hand and fingers are feeling better with less pain and numbness. Does this surprise you?

Your first treatment is a "get-acquainted" session. When you have gotten acquainted with the tissues of your forearm, you are ready to move down to your hand, fingers, and thumb.

The first thing is to simply look at your hand and fingers. Look at the skin of your palm. Is it drawn tight? Are the creases thick and deep? Does the skin have a callused appearance, as if you have done a lot of yard work? These are all indications of tissue dysfunction of an unhealthy hand. How about the fingers; do they look swollen? Are the creases at their joints thickened and deep? What about the color of your hand and fingers? Does the skin have a dark cast to it? Do the joints of your fingers have a shiny grapelike appearance? These are more indications of dysfunction.

When you straighten your thumb and fingers as far as they will go, can you feel the skin overlying your palm stretched tightly? Run your examining fingers over the surface of your hand. Does the skin feel rough?

Examine the area of your palm that lies just beyond your wrist, between the bulges of your thumb and pinky finger. Nudge this tissue with your forefinger. Does it resist? It is likely that you will find the skin here to be thick and adherent to underlying tissues. Press down on it with your examining forefinger. Does this maneuver cause increased pain and numbness in your thumb and fingers?

This is the area of the carpal tunnel! A surgeon would cut into and mutilate that tissue and charge you thousands of dollars for the disservice. You will soon find, however, that the thickened tissue can be softened and normalized, can become healthy again, by gentle, humane treatment.

Let's treat that carpal tunnel. You will be able to identify it because it will likely be thick and hard, and have a rounded surface. Apply some lotion to it. Begin the softening process with gentle nudges applied at its border. Go completely around its border with nudges that are directed toward its center. Now try thumb sweeps over the tissue. Experiment with varying amounts of lotion to get just the effect you want. Take your time.

If a surgeon has already cut into the tissue, the problem has become more complicated, but the outcome for success is still good. It will take more work, however, because you will have to soften tissue that has been surgically scarred.

Use your forefinger for circles and back-and-forths. As you work on this tissue, you are likely to experience increased pain and numbness in your thumb and fingers. These sensations are temporary. Bring the tips of your thumb and pinky finger together; this will put some slack on the carpal tunnel tissues, enabling you to knead them. Pincer and apply back-and-forths and circles. Wipe off all the lotion and repeat the previously applied movements; this will provide you with more variations and greater effect.

By this time, these tissues should have begun to soften, and you can finish the treatment here with skin ripplings. Are you pleased with the results of your treatment so far? I hope so. Do your thumb and fingers feel better?

The treatment of your hand can proceed in different directions: you can move out to the bulge of either your thumb or pinky finger. Or you might extend your palm treatment to your fingers. Once again, there is no cookbook formula. Go where your exploring fingers lead you.

Let's select the thumb. Work up the large bulge of your thumb. Use thumb probes, circles, and back-and-forths as you look for tight, hard bands that run from the joint of the bulge (at the wrist) into the thumb proper. Pincer the web of the thumb with back-and-forths and circles. Look for hard bands in there; these may be severely painful. Now go back and examine the joint at the base of the thumb bulge; this is the first thumb joint. Pincer it with your examining thumb on the palm side, and the examining forefinger opposite it (on the topside of your hand). Perform push-and-pulls. You may find excruciatingly painful areas in the joint; if so, be sure to return to treat these some time in the future. It is important to resolve joint dysfunction there.

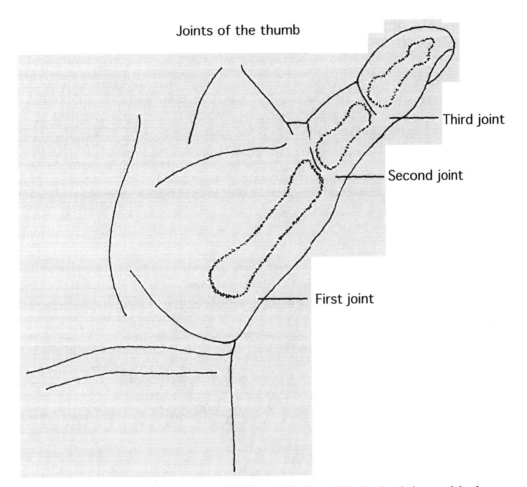

Joints of the thumb

Third joint

Second joint

First joint

Now treat the second and third thumb joints. Work the joints with the tip of your examining thumb, performing circles and back-and-forths. Look for hard, fibrotic tissue that lies deep in the joint creases.

Go back to the smaller pinky finger bulge. It is likely you will find considerably less dysfunctioning tissue than you did in the thumb bulge. Explore and treat as you did with the thumb bulge.

Now treat the skin overlying your entire palm. It will be difficult to ripple the skin because of the nature of the terrain and because the skin is likely to be tightly adherent to the tissues beneath it. Try some thumb sweeps with varying amounts of lotion. Then wipe off all the lotion and

115

perform small circles over all the skin creases; this will help to loosen the skin and free it from its adherent bonds. Then go back to thumb sweeps on the unlotioned skin. Perform the sweeps in all directions. I think you will find that your skin is now noticeably looser. Are you surprised that improvement can come so quickly?

Turn your attention to the deeper tissues of your palm, including the joints there. Pincer all joints with the tip of your examining thumb on the palm and your examining forefinger opposite, on the top of your hand. Loosen the joints with push-and-pulls, thumb probes, and circles. Alternate these maneuvers until you feel the palm joints loosening. You have likely found thick, painful tissues that prevent your palm joints from moving freely. You will be pleasantly surprised to find how quickly these tissues can soften, and your hand becomes supple and healthy again.

You are almost finished with the treatment of your hand. Treat the joints of your fingers with pincering back-and-forths and circles. Perform short thumb sweeps along all the joint creases. Try to ripple the skin overlying these creases. This will help to soften and release the skin from underlying joint structures.

Now go to the top side of your hand. Ripple the skin there. Push-pull the joints of your hand with your thumb now topside. You may find some severely painful joint tissue that will need further treatment.

Finish the treatment by going back up to your shoulder and jiggle and gently pat all the tissues from you shoulder on down to your fingertips. Enjoy the feeling of looseness and suppleness that one treatment has brought to your tissues.

Do you remember how you wiggled your fingers just before you started the treatment of your arm and hand? Now try it again, *after* treatment. Wiggle the fingers of your treated hand. Notice how much freer they are, and how quickly they move back and forth. Compare with the wiggles of your "better hand." It is likely that these cannot move as quickly; this is after just one treatment.

Continue with self-treatment sessions, and all your tissues will become soft, supple, healthy, and pain-free once again.

Chronic Pain

Doctors declare pain to be chronic when it has lasted three to six months. **Sufferers are then told it is irreversible.** They are given "pain-killers" and sent to pain management centers, the place where pain sufferers go to learn how to live with the pain they will suffer for the rest of their lives.

How sad that doctors do not understand that what they diagnose as chronic pain is a reflection of soft tissue dysfunction, and, since it is possible to treat and reverse tissue dysfunction, the resulting pain is also reversible. People do not have to suffer pain, certainly not for the rest of their lives.

Chronic pain occurs when the tissues of the body are allowed to become tight, contracted, and fibrotic. Pain will last as long as the tissue dysfunction remains untreated, whether this is three to six months, three to six years, or the entirety of the sufferer's life.

When properly treated, the early stages of tissue spasm do not develop into the later stages of contraction and fibrosis, so chronic pain will not occur. However, even the later stages of tissue dysfunction can be effectively treated and normalized, so the individual can become pain-free and healthy again.

Case History

A woman stopped by my office and asked if I could help her. She said she had been suffering severe chronic pain for eleven years. The pain had developed gradually and seemed to start a few months after a severe emotional trauma. The pain had become increasingly intense as the years passed. In addition to the excruciating pain, her body was growing stiffer, and she suffered from debilitating fatigue. She was concerned that the way things were going, she would soon end up in a wheelchair.

She told me that she also suffered from severe depression. Not only that, but because of the distracting pain, she was finding it increasingly difficult to concentrate her thoughts.

For the past few years, the pain had become unbearable. There was not a single minute she did not suffer severe body pain and headaches. She described her life as a "living hell." She had been to several doctors over the years, but none had been able to help her. All told her the same thing: "Nothing more can be done. You will have to learn to live with your pain."

But she had never given up. She had tried everything and anything that might help her: chiropractic, acupuncture, massage, herbs, yoga, meditation. Some had helped a little, some not at all. But there was always hope in the back of her mind that someday she would find something that would give her real relief.

I told her there was a possibility that I might be able to help her, but I would need a doctor's referral that would allow me to treat her. She said she would get one, and we set up an appointment.

When she came for our first session, I found that her scalp was drawn as tight as a drumhead, completely immovable, and terribly painful. As I gently palpated down her neck, I found that those tissues were intensely tender and sensitive to very light touch, as were the tissues of her entire back, abdomen, shoulders, both arms, both legs, gluteal area, and anterior trunk. Her entire body was tight, contracted, and painful.

It took me well over two hours to preliminarily check her body. Even though I was as gentle as possible, she cried out several times because of the extreme pain. I told her that, although I couldn't guarantee anything, I thought there was a chance I could help her. She said she was eager to try.

We started a healing venture that lasted a year and a half. I treated her three times a week in two to three hour sessions for the first four months. The sessions were then reduced to twice a week, then once a week, then once every two weeks, then once a month, then once every two months, until final discharge.

The first month of treatment was an agony for both of us. She cried out loudly throughout each treatment session because of the increased pain that was stirred up with even the lightest touch. I expected someone to knock on the door to see if everything was all right. Yet she continued to return for more treatment, because following each session her body was a little looser and the pain was a little less severe.

Two months after treatment started, she came in on a Monday and said that a miracle had happened over the weekend. She had gone one whole day without any pain. She considered this to be a miracle. She couldn't get over it. It was the first time in years that she had been without pain.

Thus, it continued over the next several months. Gradually, her body softened, the days without pain became more frequent, and the level of the pain diminished. Her depression began to clear, and she was able to focus her thoughts once again. She noticed that she was less fatigued.

There came a time when she no longer had any pain. All that remained was tissue tightness. We continued to work on the remaining tightness, until eventually that too was resolved. Her body was soft, supple, and free of pain. She was healthy again.

Prior to my treatments, she had been unable to work, but now she was able to get a full-time job. Her whole quality of life had changed.

When we had reduced to one treatment every two months, she became aware that at times of stress her body would begin to tighten. She learned to back away from the stress so her body wouldn't continue to tighten. A year and a half after starting, she was discharged from treatment. I told her to feel free to call me for any reason whatsoever. No call came.

I checked with her one year later. She was continuing to do fine. She did feel that she always had to be aware that stress had a tendency to retighten her body. But now that her body had been made soft and supple, she had a means of becoming aware of the first sign of retightening and was able to deal with it before it got worse.

If this woman had believed all the doctors who had told her that her chronic pain was irreversible, she never would have tried to find something that would end her pain and suffering. If she had believed her doctors, she would still be living her nightmare. It is sad that there are so many more who unfortunately do believe their doctors, and because of their misplaced trust they continue to exist in their living hell.

The Schatz Technique™ Instructions

When one suffers from what doctors call chronic pain, the entire body is usually affected. If you are one of these individuals, you have a challenging task ahead of you. I suggest that you start by examining and treating your upper extremities. Refer to "Carpal Tunnel Syndrome" for *The Schatz Technique*™ suggestions. When the tissues of your arms and hands have become normalized and free of pain, you will be better able to treat other areas of your body that may be affected.

Dizziness

Doctors associate dizziness with eye, ear, or brain disturbances. If problems in these areas cannot be found and dizziness continues, their patients are told that nothing more can be done.

However, individuals who have soft tissue problems involving the upper back, neck, and scalp may complain of dizziness. The level of dizziness can range from mild to severe. I became aware of the relationship many years ago, when patients I treated for upper back and neck pain would, from time to time, also complain of bouts of dizziness. As their soft tissue problems were resolved, their symptoms of dizziness went away. One case was particularly dramatic.

Case History

Several years ago, I was working in a large rehabilitation facility. I received a call from a physical therapy supervisor in another unit. She had just learned of a young woman who was being treated by neurologists for profound dizziness. The dizziness was so severe that the patient required the assistance of two people, one on either side, to be able to take even a few steps.

The neurologists were convinced that such severe symptoms had to be caused by a brain tumor, but after extensive and repeated tests and examinations, the tumor had not been found. Further tests were planned. The supervisor had recalled that I had mentioned to her that dizziness could be caused by soft tissue dysfunction. She said that if I were interested, she would get a referral allowing me to treat the patient.

I *was* interested, the referral *was* granted, and treatment began that afternoon. When I examined the young woman, I found that the tissues of her upper back, neck, and scalp were extremely tight, contracted, and extremely tender to mild examination. I learned that three months before her dizziness started, she had experienced a severe emotional trauma.

The patient responded rapidly to treatment. The symptoms of pain, tightness, and dizziness diminished as her tissues became softened and normalized. In two weeks, she was discharged from the facility, completely free of dizziness.

The patient responded rapidly to treatment. The symptoms of pain, tightness, and dizziness diminished as her tissues became softened and normalized. In two weeks, she was discharged from the facility, completely free of dizziness.

To my great surprise, the neurologists never contacted me to find out what I had done to so dramatically help their patient. I wonder what "other tests" they had in mind?

The Schatz Technique™ Instructions

The primary areas to be treated are the scalp, face, neck, and upper back. Review "Migraine and Muscle Contraction Headaches," and treat as indicated.

Dowager's Hump

"Dowager's hump" is a lay term describing the unsightly hump of tissue overlying the spinal column at the upper back that one sees occasionally on women of varying age. The hump is not caused by a distortion of the vertebrae, and is usually dismissed by doctors–if it is noticed at all–as being nothing more than an accumulation of fat.

However, if this tissue is properly examined, it will be found to be composed of thickened, contracted, and fibrotic tissue. The skin overlying this area is thick, painful, and adherent to underlying tissues. If the tissues above, below, and to either side of the hump are palpated, they also will be found to be contracted, fibrotic, and painful.

In other words, a dowager's hump is really an area of soft tissue dysfunction and, furthermore, it is an indication that there are other extensive areas of soft tissue dysfunction. It is important that the dysfunctioning tissue of a dowager's hump be treated and normalized along with the extensive areas that contributed to its formation.

Patients do not come to me with dowager's hump as a presenting symptom. It is more of a flag, an indicator, of global dysfunction. Therefore, a case history for dowager's hump will not be presented.

The Schatz Technique™

The Schatz Technique™ **Instructions**

Treatment consists of normalizing the tissues associated with it: the neck, upper and mid-back, and both upper extremities. For *The Schatz Technique™* suggestions refer to "Migraines and Muscle Contraction Headaches" and "Carpal Tunnel Syndrome."

It is important before beginning self-treatment to see a physician in order to rule out any vertebral problem.

Dupuytren's Contracture

Dupuytren's contracture is a progressive disorder of the hand in which a nodule forms in the palm, and the fingers are gradually pulled tightly onto the palm. The individual is unable to straighten them, and it becomes increasingly difficult to use the hand in a normal manner.

Dupuytren's contracture does not respond well to drugs, stretching or exercise. Surgery is crude and results in the formation of scar tissue and possible nerve damage. The hand is unable to perform precise movements. If the individual is unfortunate enough to be a musician, a change of careers is very likely.

Case History

A woman called and said she had Dupuytren's contracture. Her doctor told her surgery would be required. She had heard of my work and wondered if I might be able to help her avoid surgery. I told her to get a referral that would allow me to examine and treat, and we set up an appointment.

The Schatz Technique™

When I examined her, I found the characteristic nodule in the palm of her right hand, and noted that three of her fingers were curled tightly. She was unable to straighten them. I also noted tight, contracted tissues throughout both upper extremities.

She responded well to treatment. The nodule rapidly softened, and in six weeks all tissues were supple and healthy. When discharged from treatment, the nodule was completely gone and she could extend all fingers freely and easily.

The Schatz Technique™ **Instructions**

For appropriate suggestions for *The Schatz Technique™* , refer to "Carpal Tunnel Syndrome."

Ear Pain

Ear pain can be caused by a number of problems, infectious to neurologic. At times, even though doctors have explored and ruled out every possible source known to them, the patient continues to suffer. The pain of these individuals is likely caused by soft tissue dysfunction.

Case History

I received a call from a woman who said her seventy-three-year old mother was suffering excruciating pain in her left ear. It was so severe and distracting that her mother could no longer use her walker to get about. The pain had continued over a three-week period. Her mother had been examined by several doctors, including an ear, nose, and throat specialist, and a neurologist, but the cause of pain had not been discovered.

The caller had heard of my work and wondered if I could help. I told her I would need a doctor's consent that would allow me to examine and treat her mother. She said she would obtain one, and we set up an appointment. Because her mother was so incapacitated by her pain, I agreed to treat her at their home.

When I arrived for the first treatment, I found the patient seated in a chair with her head tilted to the left. She was cradling her head in her left hand and was moaning with pain.

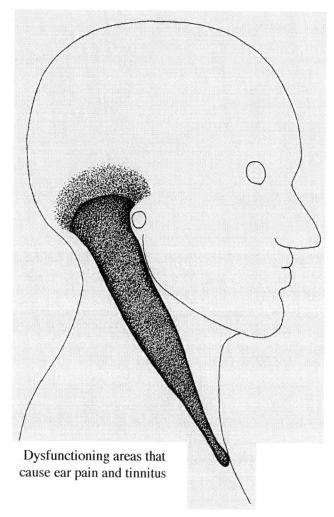

Dysfunctioning areas that cause ear pain and tinnitus

I found that her scalp was drawn tight and was painful to light examination. The tissues of her face were thickened and fibrotic, as were the tissues at her upper back (i.e., the trapezius muscle). But most involved were the muscles at the front of her neck, the sternocleidomastoids. The left one was more affected than the right, particularly where it attached just behind her left ear. At the point of attachment, it was hard, thick, and fibrotic. Touching the area lightly caused her to cry out and to hold her head more guardedly.

I worked on the affected tissues with great care, and as I did so, the pain eased and her body relaxed. I treated her three times a week until I discharged her two weeks later. At that time, she no longer experienced any pain, and the tight and contracted tissues had softened significantly.

What was thought to be pain *in* her ear was really pain caused by soft tissue dysfunction *close to* her ear. When this was properly treated, the pain went away.

The Schatz Technique™ **Instructions**

The primary area of soft tissue dysfunction that underlies ear pain is where the sternocleidomastoid muscle attaches just behind the ear. Other areas of soft tissue dysfunction that likely contribute to ear pain are the scalp, face, neck and upper back.

Lie on your back with your head comfortably supported by pillows. Arrange them so your head is tilted forward, this will produce some slack in your sternocleidomastoids. Let us assume that your left ear is the painful one. You will turn your head to the left; this will further relax the muscle where it attaches behind your left ear.

Slip your right hand under your head so the palm of your hand supports the weight of your head. This will free your fingers and thumb to explore and treat. Start your treatment at the area of attachment with your first and second fingers held closely together, i.e., doubled. This makes them into a very effective probing instrument. Use them to perform circles and back-and-forths. Take your time; don't rush. Treat the entire area that surrounds your ear, paying particular attention to the tissue behind and below.

Are you finding thick tissue that becomes painful with gentle treatment? Move up into the scalp region. Let your fingers follow any pain or contracted areas. As you move outward, add multiple finger movements.

Go back to the attachment and examine the sternocleidomastoid itself. Move down and pincer it gently between thumb and bent forefinger as you go. Roll it gently, feeling for contracted, fibrotic or painful areas. Try some gentle single-finger circles, back-and-forths, and single-finger stationary presses. Move down to where the muscle attaches to the chest wall and examine and treat. Use single-finger, double-finger, and multiple-finger circles.

Explore and treat the tissues of your face. Let your fingers look for tight, contracted areas and for areas that cause any increase of your ear pain. For treatment of the upper back, refer to "Migraine and Muscle Contraction Headaches."

Examine and treat the skin overlying all the tissue areas you treated. Pay particular attention to the skin overlying the attachment of the sternocleidomastoid. You will undoubtedly find it thickened and painful. Notice how thick the skin is as it blends into your ear. Use your thumb for skin ripples and circles. Treat thoroughly.

Dysfunctioning tissues that underlie ear pain may have been developing for a long period of time (years) before symptoms become apparent. Accordingly, these tissues may not respond quickly, and will require patient and diligent care to soften and normalize them so the pain will go away and stay away.

Emotional Pain

(Expressed with Panic Attacks, Sleep

Disorders, Depression, Agoraphobia)

When an individual experiences trauma, physical or emotional, body tissues tighten and contract and are, in effect, imprinted with that stress or trauma. Just as the tissues of the face reflect emotional stress, so do the tissues of the rest of the body. Once an emotional signal has been translated into a physical form, the imprinted physical component is now capable of recycling the signals, causing increasing emotional distress, as well as physical pain and physical dysfunction.

I have treated women who told me they had been sexually abused. All developed profound physical pain and dysfunction that was challenging to treat, in addition to their continuing emotional problems. I suspect that all victims of sexual abuse, and other severe emotional trauma, require soft tissue treatment to reverse and normalize the physical imprint (in addition to whatever psychotherapy they may be receiving) to achieve maximum healing. Attempting to treat a serious emotional problem without treating the physical component renders a disservice to the patient. The present-day psychiatric practitioner is apparently unaware of this.

There is a flip side to this. When an individual has been insulted by physical trauma, i.e. bodily injury, there frequently is a resulting emotional component, that is to say, an emotional overlay. In other words, both physical and emotional trauma can produce emotional symptoms. These can take the form of panic attacks, sleep disorder, depression, and agoraphobia. The patient in the following case history experienced all of these symptoms.

Case History

A woman in her fifties was referred for treatment of a severely painful shoulder. Her doctor informed me that because of "emotional problems" she was unable to leave her home, and I would have to treat her there. I phoned her and set up an appointment.

When I met with her, I learned that she had been injured in a car accident when she was five years old. She had also sustained very severe emotional trauma at an early age. Throughout the ensuing years, her body was plagued with pain and tightness and she suffered from severe headaches.

She also experienced emotional problems, depression, sleep disorders, and panic attacks, and she had recently been diagnosed as having agoraphobia (fear of being in a crowd or public place). She was aware that her physical and emotional problems were growing worse. Medications and psychological counseling had not helped. She lost her job because of these problems, and she said she was at the end of her strength.

When I examined her, I found that the tissues of her entire body were tight, contracted, fibrotic, and painful. Her shoulder was hurting, but so was the rest of her body. Her scalp, face, neck, and upper back were particularly tight and painful to light examination.

After the first treatment, she said she felt more relaxed than she had for a long time. When I returned to give her a second treatment, she said that her body was still hurting but she had slept "a little better." As treatments continued, her physical pain and emotional problems became less severe. Two to three hours of fitful sleep was all she could attain when treatment started, but she gradually experienced deeper sleep for longer periods.

I treated her in two-hour sessions, three times a week for two weeks, then twice a week for two weeks. I was then able to reduce treatment to once a week for one month, then down to once every two weeks for a total of five months.

Because her problems were of such long duration–over fifty years–we were not able to achieve a complete recovery. However, when she was discharged at the end of five months, her condition had significantly improved. She could have five to six hours of refreshing sleep. Her emotional problems had lessened, and she was able to leave her house and start working again. She was extremely pleased with the results of the treatments.

The Schatz Technique™ Instructions

The areas of soft tissue dysfunction that are associated with emotional pain can occur anywhere in the body. Frequently, they are the same areas that generate headaches, that is, the scalp, face, neck, upper back, and chest. Refer to the headache section "Migraine and Muscle Contraction Headaches" for treatment suggestions. You may have to explore your body for other tissue areas that underlie your problem.

Fibromyalgia

Or;

There's a Bridge For Sale In Brooklyn That You Might Want to Buy

Doctors invented an impressive-sounding word to, well, impress their patients--when their patients complain of muscle pain. That word is...."fibromyalgia."

You see, "myalgia" *means* "muscle pain." So, when patients suffering muscle pain are told by their doctors that they have fibromyalgia, they are merely being told that they have muscle pain--something they already knew. Indeed, that is why they went to their doctors in the first place.

Patients would not be impressed with their doctors' intelligence if they went to them complaining of muscle pain, and their doctors said "yes, you have muscle pain." But they are greatly impressed when their doctors tell them: you have "fibromyalgia."

Doctors also invented an impressive-sounding method of producing a "diagnosis" of fibromyalgia. Impressive-sounding, yes, but when examined, turns out to be complex, confusing, and worthless. Judge for yourself:

Doctors produce a diagnosis of fibromyalgia using a combination of two criteria as directed by "**The American College of Rheumatology Criteria for the Classification of Fibromyalgia:**"

1. **Pain throughout the body**. "Pain throughout the body" is not a useful basis of diagnosis.

2. **Pain in eleven of eighteen tender point sites**. Here is where things get interesting, because it does *sound* scientific. However, let's look a

little closer. Medical literature tells us it is important that a "tender point" *cannot be tender*, it must be painful. If it is tender, not painful, when pressed upon, then it is not a countable tender point. (Are you keeping up with this)?

How does the doctor know if a site is "tender, not painful" or, "painful, not tender?" **He asks the patient.**

Everyone has an individual perception of pain. One person might describe a particular stimulus as "painful," while another person might describe an identical level of stimulus as "tender." This well known phenomenon means the entire premise that "pain in eleven of eighteen tender point sites" demonstrates that someone "has" fibromyalgia, is nonsense.

Hold on, there's more:

Since the individual has "pain all over" as expressed in criterion number one (of the "Rheumatology College"), it is likely that she will have pain wherever she is pressed. To meet this dilemma, doctors present us with a point they say is "less likely to be painful when pressed." They call this additional point a "control point."

If someone states they have pain in more than three control points, the doctor says she does not have fibromyalgia (even if she has those eleven of eighteen tender points, that is, painful tender points). And what, you might ask, if a patient has only ten (not the "magic" number of eleven) painful tender points? What does *she* have? Ask a doctor, ask **YOUR** doctor.

Doctors have given a name to yet another point they might accidentally press upon while they are busily pressing on all those other points. They call this point a "trigger point." When pressing on a patient to differentiate between painful, tender, tender (not painful), and control points, the doctor must be on the alert not to confuse the trigger point with any of *those* other points. You see, trigger points can be be both painful *and* tender ("painful" in one place and "tender" in another), but doctors feel they are not related to what they call "fibromyalgia."

Fibromyalgia still sounding scientific?

Doctors need to press on all those various points on all parts of their patients' bodies with exactly the same amount of pressure as other doctors throughout the country, in order to convince us that this is truly a "scientific examination technique."

In order to solve *this* dilemma, doctors came up with the novel idea that this uniform pressure is the amount of pressure it takes to blanche a doctor's thumbnail. Which means that all thumbnails throughout the country, big, small, thick, thin, young, old, blunt, pointy, all blanche to the same degree when pressing on those many points.

The sad thing is that even if pressing on all those points led to reproducible results, doctors still wouldn't know what is *causing* those points to become painful or tender, or *why* their patients hurt all over and are so fatigued.

Doctors do not understand that contracted skin, fascia, muscles, and ligaments can squeeze pain receptors, blood vessels, and nerves, thereby causing the symptoms of pain and fatigue to which they have affixed the hollow word of fibromyalgia.

Since doctors do not understand the cause of what they call fibromyalgia, they do not know how to treat that cause. As a result of their ignorance, they declare that "fibromyalgia" is incurable, and attempt to manage the symptoms with drugs, exercise, and diet.

Individuals diagnosed as having fibromyalgia have called from time to time asking if I could help them. I told them I would need a doctor's referral in order to examine and treat them. In all cases, their doctors refused to sign one.

The Schatz Technique™ Instructions

I have successfully treated individuals such as the patient mentioned in the chronic pain section, who experienced similar symptoms as those having "fibromyalgia."

If you have been "diagnosed" as having fibromyalgia, you probably suffer from extensive areas of soft tissue dysfunction and have a lot of work ahead of you.

My treatment suggestions are the same that I offer in the section on "chronic pain."

Start by examining and treating your upper extremities. Refer to "Carpal Tunnel Syndrome" for instructions for *The Schatz Technique™*. When the tissues of your arms and hands have become normalized and free of pain, you will be better able to treat other areas of your body that may be affected.

NEWS FLASH!

FDA APPROVES ELI LILLY'S CYMBALTA FOR "TREATMENT" OF FIBROMYALGIA

A few comments:

I. The FDA approval of Cymbalta for "Treatment" of fibromyalgia was based on "clinical trials" that included a very small number of participants **(only 874)** for an extremely short test period **(only three months!)**.

--Do you trust the FDA for approving a drug with a small number of participants for a short test period, and for saying that it "treats" Fibromyalgia when it really doesn't? The drug not directed toward those eleven of eighteen tender point sites that doctors tell us is the cause of "Fibromyalgia." (Cymbalta is an antidepressant!)
 Why would the FDA do such a terrible thing to a trusting public? Seems to me that some sort of fraud might be involved here. This needs looking into.

2. Eli Lilly previously **pleaded guilty** to a **criminal count** of violating the Food, Drug and Cosmetic Act by off-label marketing of another of its drugs. It paid $36 million in fines in connection with its **illegal promotion** of its pharmaceutical drug Evista.

--Do you trust <u>anything</u> this company now says about Cymbalta?

3. In the "clinical trials," Cymbalta was compared with a placebo ("sugar pills") and even with this non-contest, the "results" were minimal. Keep in mind the drug **doesn't treat** fibromyalgia. **The drug is designed to produce psychogenic changes.**

--Do you want to take a drug that fools around with your brain?

4. Cymbalta is an antidepressant that can have *horrendous* side-effects, such as **liver damage that can lead to death**, and **thoughts of suicide** that can lead to **actual suicide**. It can also cause a myriad number of extremely unpleasant side-effects such as "worsening of depression symptoms, unusual changes in behavior, anxiety, agitation, panic attacks, difficulty sleeping, irritability, hostility, aggressiveness, impulsivity, restlessness, or extreme hyperactivity." And once you start taking the drug, you can have a devil of a time trying to get off it.

--Do you think its worth all these risks to take a drug that doesn't really treat fibromyalgia?

137

Frozen Shoulder

Frozen shoulder, a painful and disabling problem, is ill defined and misunderstood by the medical community. The attention of doctors is focused at the point of the patient's complaint of pain: the shoulder joint. The problem, however, usually lies with contracted soft tissue well away from the joint. The medical profession is unaware that pain *perceived* to be inside a joint invariably radiates from dysfunctioning tissues outside the joint.

The upper extremity is connected to the torso primarily by muscles that are attached close to the shoulder joint. However, some of these muscles are large, and their torso origin is far from the shoulder. The latissimus dorsi, for example, originates *as far away as the pelvis*.

If these muscles become contracted, the shoulder is not allowed to move freely. If severely contracted, they hold the shoulder tightly against the torso. The shoulder becomes "frozen." The problem is not with the shoulder joint, but with the contracted muscles attached to the shoulder area.

The proper treatment for a "frozen shoulder," therefore, is to soften and normalize these muscles and their associated tissues. When this is done, the shoulder moves freely again.

Case History 1

The patient I am about to discuss was treated very early in my career. Her case was pivotal in pointing me toward recognizing the global aspect of soft tissue dysfunction. She was a woman in her sixties, referred to me when I was a staff physical therapist at a rehabilitation center.

She had a painfully frozen shoulder that had developed gradually over a two-year period, but the cause was unknown. Her shoulder had become excruciatingly painful three months before I saw her.

At the time, I knew little about soft tissue dysfunction. I had been taught that to treat a frozen shoulder, you applied moist heat to the shoulder joint, followed by ultrasound to the shoulder joint, followed by stretching of the shoulder joint. The stretching was performed both manually and with the aid of a "shoulder wheel," which produced an effect that must have been similar to what stretching a victim on the rack in the Dark Ages must have produced: intense and excruciating pain. I proceeded to practice what I had been taught, but when I attempted to stretch her shoulder, she cried out in pain. Being softhearted, I stopped.

The only thing I could think to do for her was to reach out and gently touch her painful shoulder to try to soothe it. It was a natural act of compassion rather than a treatment technique. However, this seemed to give her some relief, so I started to gently massage her shoulder and arm. She felt a little better at the end of the session, so another was scheduled.

This continued for several weeks. Gradually, her pain eased and the tightness around her shoulder softened. As those tissues softened, I became aware that tissues farther away from her shoulder were also tight, contracted, and painful. I began to work on those areas.

I found myself gradually working down her upper arm, forearm, and wrist. Two months into treatment I was able to work on painful tissues in her hand and fingers, the last areas that needed treatment. Suddenly she remembered what had started the whole problem.

Two years earlier, a few months before she noticed pain in her shoulder, a purse had been snatched from her. In the struggle, two of her fingers had become injured and painful. The relationship between her injured fingers and her frozen shoulder had not occurred to her until I began to work on them and the remaining pain had jogged her memory.

It was only after, and because, we had persistently tracked and released the tissue from her shoulder, down through her arm, forearm, hand and fingers, that the connection was made. I figured the soft tissues had gradually tightened, somehow, from her injured finger on up to her shoulder.

The light was turned on. The global aspect and inter-connectedness of soft tissue dysfunction was revealed. A problem starting in a finger caused a problem in a shoulder. What this said to me was that a problem starting in any part of the body can cause a problem in any other part of the body, no matter how distant from each other the parts happen to be. Injure one part of the body, and eventually the entire body may become affected.

Case History 2

A woman in her early seventies came for treatment of a severely painful frozen shoulder. She had fractured her left humerus (the bone of the upper arm) six months earlier, and during the course of the healing, her shoulder had become frozen.

She had already received intensive physical therapy as prescribed by her doctor. The physical therapy consisted of hot packs, ultrasound, and stretching exercises to the shoulder joint. In addition, her doctor had injected cortisone into the shoulder joint. However, despite a long course of the above treatments, her shoulder had become increasingly painful and even more frozen.

She had heard of my work and had obtained a doctor's referral that allowed me to treat her. Unfortunately, her doctor's referral called for more of the same treatment already proven to be ineffective, namely, more hot packs, more ultrasound, and more stretching exercises. I called the doctor's office and was successful, after some difficulty, in having the order changed to "evaluate and treat," which allowed me to work in the manner I thought best.

The Schatz Technique™

When I examined the patient, I found that she had lost fifty percent of her shoulder movement. When she tried to move past the end point of her range of motion, she experienced severe pain at the shoulder. When I palpated her tissues, I found that the muscles and tissues outside her shoulder joint were tight, spasmed, contracted, and very painful to the touch. She was surprised that we were finding so many painful areas well away from her shoulder, some as far away as her lower back.

She responded well to treatment. By the end of her first two hour treatment, she had gained an additional twenty percent of shoulder motion. I treated her daily for one week. Treatments were reduced to three times a week the following week, then to two times the next week. The next week was a one-time check-over.

At the time of discharge, four weeks after start of care, she had full range of motion, without any pain, and she was a very happy lady. A follow-up call two months later revealed she remained pain and symptom-free; an additional call one year later, she was still pain- and symptom-free.

Of course I sent reports of my treatments to her doctor, but I received no response or inquiries from him as to what I had done for his patient that had caused her dramatic improvement.

The Schatz Technique™ Instructions

The primary areas of soft tissue dysfunction that contribute to so-called frozen shoulder are: (1) upper extremity; (2) chest; (3) upper back; and (4) mid to low back (latissimus dorsi muscle and associated tissues).

Treat the tissues of your upper extremity first. Refer to "Carpal Tunnel Syndrome" for *The Schatz Technique™* instructions.

Now treat your chest area. Refer to "Treating your chest" in the section titled "Migraine and Muscle Contraction Headaches."

Then treat your upper to lower back tissues. For *The Schatz Technique™* instructions for the upper back, refer to "Treating your neck and upper back" in "Migraine and Muscle Contraction Headaches." For the lower back, refer to "Back Pain."

Hip Pain and

Degenerative Joint Disease

Doctors believe that joints degenerate because of disease intrinsic to the joint itself, that is why they characterize the problem as a "joint disease." Doctors do not carefully examine the bodies of their patients and therefore do not understand that joint dysfunction is primarily caused by the prolonged stress of contracted body tissues *outside* the joint.

A joint is stressed when the tissues surrounding it become tight and contracted. If this stress continues over a protracted period, the structure of the joint begins to change, to degenerate. If this process is allowed to continue for years, the joint may become so damaged that it eventually has to be replaced with a metal and plastic one.

Fortunately, nature provides us with the early warning system of pain. Pain alerts the individual that something is wrong. The proper response of doctors would be to carefully examine the body to find what is causing the alarm signal of pain. Tight, contracted tissues would then be identified and treated, the sensation of pain would go away, as well as the stress to the joint, and the joint would remain healthy. Sadly, doctors do not heed the alarm signal of pain; in fact, believe it or not, they actually attempt to kill it with pain-killers. The growth of the extremely lucrative mechanical-joint industry continues at an alarming rate.

Case History

The histories of several patients I have treated over the years indicate that difficult birthings, and even not-so-difficult birthings, can contribute significantly to soft tissue dysfunction, which in turn causes the joints of the body to become dysfunctional. I recall one woman in particular whose case illustrates this.

This woman noticed pain in her hips a few months after a difficult birth. As years went on, her knees also became painful. The pain gradually became severe and constant, and was accompanied by increasing tightness of her hips and knees. She was given pain-killing drugs, muscle relaxants, and cortisone injections, without any effect on either the pain or tightness.

I saw her thirty-four years after that difficult birth. As a matter of fact, it was my questioning about her early history that elicited her recollection about it and the ensuing pain and tightness. This had not been explored by any of the doctors who had treated her.

By the time soft tissue treatment was started, so many years following the onset of her problem, I was able to provide her with only limited improvement. The tissues on her right side were successfully released and became pain-free, but the joint structures of her left hip and knee were so damaged by the continued stress of contracted tissue for such a long period of time that I suggested she talk to her doctor about joint replacements.

This was done, and she became relatively pain-free. It is tragic that she suffered pain for so many years and eventually was subjected to drastic surgical joint replacement when timely soft tissue treatment likely would have prevented her problems.

The Schatz Technique™ **Instructions**

Any joint in the body can be stressed by tight and contracted body tissues. If you suffer pain perceived to be coming from a joint, and intrinsic joint problems such as rheumatoid arthritis have been ruled out, and your doctor is talking about *replacing* your joint with a mechanical one, it would be wise to see if you can solve your problem with self-treatment. Refer to the appropriate symptom area that relates to where you are hurting. If you are experiencing hip pain, refer to "Back Pain." Also refer to treatment of "The Knee" (Tensor Fascia Lata) under "Knee Pain," as this structure is a frequent contributor to hip joint pain.

Knee Pain

FTH: (Frequently The Hamstrings)

Doctors attempt to treat knee pain with pain-killing drugs, surgery and the replacement of natural joints with mechanical ones. However, knee pain is frequently caused by contracted tissues *outside* the knee joint. The pain is *referred* to the inside of the joint. Although the sufferer can swear the pain is inside the joint, it actually radiates from exterior tissues.

Knee pain is frequently caused by dysfunctioning Hamstrings. These are the muscles and associated tissues that bend our knees. Hamstrings are often contracted, thickened and fibrotic. I believe Hamstrings become severely affected because we spend so much time sitting with our knees bent for extended periods. This prolonged "bent position" sets the Hamstrings up for development of tissue dysfunction.

As the years roll on, Hamstrings become more and more dysfunctional. I suspect that dysfunctional Hamstrings, ignored by doctors, lead to large numbers of unnecessary knee replacements.

Other important causes of knee pain will be discussed in this section. Proper treatment is to normalize the tight and contracted tissues that are radiating pain and causing stress to the knee joint. When this is done pain will go away and the knee remains healthy.

146

Mechanical joint replacement is becoming increasingly popular these days. Indeed, mechanical joint replacement can be a blessing in eliminating the excruciating pain of severe joint dysfunction. The tragedy is that, often as not, the need for mechanical joint replacement can be entirely avoided, along with years of agonizing pain.

It takes a long period of time for the tight, contracted, and fibrotic tissues that surround a joint to eventually stress the structures of that joint to become so dysfunctional that it must be replaced with one made of metal and plastic. During all those years, there are progressive alarm signals of pain that cry out for help. If doctors knew how to interpret those alarm signals and to properly respond to them, they could save their patients years of pain and the eventuality of drastic and mutilating surgery.

Knee pain is frequently caused by dysfunctioning Hamstrings. These are the muscles and associated tissues that bend our knees. Hamstrings are often contracted, thickened, and fibrotic. As the years roll on, Hamstrings become more and more dysfunctional.

Case History 1

A woman was referred for treatment of a painful shoulder. When I chatted with her, I learned she was a retired surgical nurse. She was forced to accept early retirement fourteen years early because of a terribly painful right knee. Standing on hard floors for many years had apparently caused the knee problem. During her years of retirement, she continued to suffer severe, agonizing pain.

I asked if anything had been done to help her knee pain. She said doctors had tried everything, but nothing had helped. Her orthopedic doctor told her the *only* thing that would end her pain was a mechanical knee replacement. She declined this procedure because of her experiences as a surgical nurse.

I told her there was a chance I would be able to help her painful knee. I called her doctor and received permission to try. We decided to split the treatment into two parts: first, we would work on her shoulder, then we would work on her knee.

Her shoulder responded quickly to treatment, well within an hour. When I examined the tissues of her right leg, I found there was extensive tissue dysfunction, from her hip on down to her calf. Wherever I touched, I found tight, contracted, and fibrotic tissue. Particularly affected was her tensor fascia lata.

I worked on those tissues for an hour. When I felt they had loosened somewhat, I told her she could get down from the treatment table and we would see if she was any better. She got down and began to bend her knee back and forth. "This is a miracle," she said. "It doesn't hurt; it absolutely doesn't hurt."

She said she would be right back and hurriedly left the office. After a few moments, she returned. She had been *running* up and down the stairs. For years she had to hobble painfully up and down stairs with a stiff leg. She couldn't wait to get home and tell her son what had happened.

When she returned for a follow-up visit two days later, she reported she was continuing to feel fine, with no return of pain. When I examined her tissues, I found there were still significant contracted areas.

I gave her two more treatments. The contracted areas were slow to respond, but she continued to remain pain-free. I suggested that, since she was doing so well, we try to see how she would do without further treatment, but to call me at the first sign of return of pain.

We kept in touch, and there was no return of pain. Two years after treatment, she called and told me she had something that would be of great interest to me.

She had been back to her orthopedic doctor for another matter, and in the course of the visit she asked if he recalled her painful knee and the necessity of a total knee replacement. He said he certainly did recall it. She then showed him how she could move her knee without any pain or discomfort. He asked, "Who did this to you?" She told him a "wonderful" (her word) physical therapist, Bernard Schatz. I asked what he then said. Her reply was "nothing."

148

I last heard from her a few months later. She continued to feel fine. She was about to go on an ocean cruise and called to thank me for helping her and changing her life so much. Naturally, that made me feel wonderful.

By the way, I never heard from her orthopedic doctor. I thought he would have had enough professional interest to find out what I had done so he could use the information to help his other patients avoid having their natural joints replaced by mechanical ones, but I guess he didn't.

Case History 2

A dentist friend frequently complained of severe pain in his left knee. The pain started a few years earlier after he had injured his knee during martial arts practice. His complaints continued for over a year. I told him I would be glad to take a look and see if there was something I could do to help. He said no, his knee had already been examined by an orthopedic doctor, and the only thing that could help was surgery.

He continued to decline my offer to see if there was anything I could do. His thought was that the pain was coming from inside the knee joint, and there was nothing I could do to help a problem coming from *inside* the knee by working on the tissues *outside*. He felt the only thing that could possibly help him was surgical intervention, which he wanted to avoid as long as possible.

I told him that frequently when someone is certain that pain is coming from within a joint, it actually is being referred from outside the joint. He remained firm in his conviction that the problem was dysfunction inside the knee.

One day, however, he called to say his knee was so excruciatingly painful that he was willing to see if there was something I could do to help him, even if just a little. I told him to get a doctor's referral and I would see him.

When I examined him, I found the tissues of his thigh from his hip down were contracted. His tissues responded well. I could feel them soften as I worked on them. After an hour, they had softened appreciably. I told him he could get off the treatment table and see how his knee felt. He got down, put some weight on his leg, bent his knee, walked around the office, and announced that he had no pain whatsoever. That was eight years ago. His knee has remained pain-free since that one treatment.

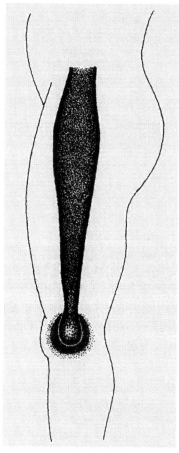

A primary cause of knee pain and dysfunction is the "Knee Destroyer" (tensor fascia lata) that runs down the outer thigh. After years of gradual tightening and pain, it damages the knee joint to such an extent that the joint has to be replaced with a metal and plastic one. Timely soft tissue work avoids this drastic surgery.

Case History 3

A woman in her sixties called to see if I could help her. She had received an artificial knee joint three months earlier but continued to experience severe knee pain. She complained to the surgeon who had performed the joint replacement, but he had dismissed her complaints of pain.

When I examined her, I found that the tissues above her knee were swollen and painful to light touch. I treated them gently, and when the swelling subsided, contracted tissues were revealed. These responded to treatment, and in one month she was discharged, pain-free.

She was pleased with the results of treatment, and did not question the need for her joint replacement, or how it could be that she was able to experience pain in a knee joint that was now a mechanical one. I left those matters undiscussed.

The Schatz Technique™ Instructions

(**As mentioned throughout this book, doctors are not trained to properly examine and treat <u>soft tissue</u> problems. However, they are trained to detect other kinds of problems, such as cancer, for example--so it is important that you have your pain checked out by a doctor to rule out things they understand.**

A particular word of caution: before self-treating your leg, have your doctor rule out a serious, life threatening condition called "deep vein thrombosis.")

Knee pain is primarily caused by tissue dysfunction above the knee: contracted thigh muscles and their associated tissues (skin and fascia) that stress their attachment points. The muscle group at the <u>front</u> of the thigh (the quadriceps) straightens the knee. The muscles at the <u>back</u> of the thigh (the hamstrings) bend the knee. Then there is the tensor fascia lata, a knee stabilizer. It runs down the <u>outer border</u> of the thigh. All of these tissues have attachment points on the shin bone, about an inch *beyond* the knee joint.

This attachment area is where knee pain is usually generated. However, the pain radiates, and is thought to be coming from *inside* the knee joint. Exploring the tissues with lotion is required to find the precise points of pain--and to normalize them. Also, keep in mind that it is the contracted tissues up in the thigh that are tightly pulling on these attachment points. Those tissues also have to be located and normalized.

You need to purchase a stool (inexpensive plastic ones are available). Get yourself into a comfortable sitting position. Let's assume your right knee is the painful one. Place a towel under your thigh, and a pillow on the footstool. Put your foot on the pillow and push the stool away a bit (you will be adjusting the position of the stool, back and forth, from time to time, to get just the right amount of slack in the particular tissues you are treating).

We'll start with the "attachment area" and work upwards. Apply some lotion on your shin bone, an inch or two beyond your knee. Place your thumbs on the top of the knee cap of your bent knee. This will put your fingers at just about the right place to explore those attachments. Have your fingers explore with small circles--then larger ones. Use the tips of your fingers (fingernails need to be closely clipped).

Explore with back and forths. Let the lotion dry a bit, so you can use the added friction to move the skin over the deeper tissues--this will help you locate points that are generating pain, and also help soften them. Look for little "b-b's," or things that feel like "wires"--anything that generates pain." Tissue dysfunction can take many forms. Now dip your fingers in the cup of water, and explore with the lotion made more slippery. This will add a helpful variation to your exploring.

When you find something that generates pain, *continue* gently exploring it--don't "rub" or "massage" it. Exploring provides <u>just the right amount</u> of interaction with dysfunctioning tissues that allows them to relax and become healthy and pain free.

151

Keep moving the stool back and forth. This will bend and straighten your knee. Notice how this loosens or tightens the tissues you are exploring. This variation of looseness and tightness will help you find hidden pain areas. When you are exploring (treating) tissues that straightens your knee (those at the top of your thigh as you look down on) it is best to have your knee in a straightened position. When exploring tissues that bend the knee, it is best to have the knee in a more bent position. Try it, and see if you agree.

I'd wager that as you explored the tissues <u>beyond</u> your knee, you found areas that surprised you by the amount of pain they generated--and how the pain lessened, or completely went away as you explored.

Now explore the tissues <u>above</u> your knee. Start with the tissues around your kneecap. Completely straighten your knee and rest the palms of your hands on top of your thigh. Using the tips of your fingers move/explore the tissues surrounding your kneecap. With your knee straight, you should be able to move your kneecap from side to side, and up and down. If you find that your kneecap is bound down by thickened tissues, you need to explore and normalize those tissues.

Continue working upwards. With your thumbs close together and your palms resting on the top of your thigh, use your fingers to explore the tissues at the top of your thigh. Have them make little circles, back-and-forths and other exploring variations described in the Glossary on page 49. Continue exploring until you reach your hip.

Go back to your kneecap. This time, keep your fingers stationary and use your thumbs to explore, from kneecap to hip joint. Repeat this sequence several times. First using fingers, then thumbs to explore. Feel free to go back and re-explore the tissues beyond your knee. This is your very first treatment, you will continue to re-explore tissues in future treatments, until your tissues are completely healthy and your knee pain is a thing of the past.

Now let's explore the tissues at the back of your thigh (the bottom as you look down). These are your hamstrings. Tight, contracted hamstrings are frequently a source of severe knee pain and dysfunction. If you experience increased pain after sitting awhile, you probably have dysfunctioning hamstrings.

By the way, have you noticed, over the years, that your knees have become increasingly "fat?" It is likely that what you have mistaken for fat, is really those pesky hamstrings. Try this: apply some lotion to those "fat tissues" at the sides of your knee, and explore. If you find hidden pain in those tissues, you have a hamstring problem that needs to be addressed.

You have to explore and normalize any dysfunctioning hamstring tissues. Bring that stool toward you--so your knee is bent, and place your thumbs on the top of your thigh. This will put your fingers underneath your thigh-just where you want them to explore your hamstrings. Be sure you have a towel under you--to prevent lotion from getting on your chair or sofa.

Explore the tissues underneath your thigh, from knee to hip. Repeat several times. Now, move your thumbs down to your fingers, so you can grasp the tissues between thumb and fingers. Move the grasped tissue in circles and back and forths. You will likely find thick, painful tissues the closer you get to the attachment area. This is where the false-fat areas occur.

Bring your thumb toward your fingers to ripple the skin. Do you find a lot of hidden pain in what you thought was fat? The more you explore, the healthier and less painful these tissues become--and your knees will get slimmer and slimmer.

Straighten your knee--this will reveal to your exploring fingers/thumb how contracted your hamstrings have become, and why you have so much pain and difficulty straightening your legs when you go to stand after sitting awhile. Follow the hamstrings as they go beyond your knee. This will lead you to the "attachment area," where you will once again reexplore.

You have now had your first session of exploring and treating the tissues that straighten and bend your knee.

You are ready to begin normalizing the tensor fascia lata--the "knee destroyer." I have given it this name because it made up of extremely tough, strong fascia. And, when this tough fascia becomes contracted, it pulls on the knee joint with a large amount of torque. If stress is allowed to continue for an extended number of years, the integrity of the knee joint is eventually destroyed.

To treat the tensor fascia lata of your right leg, you need to lie on your left side. Apply some lotion to the outside of your thigh, <u>up by your hip joint</u> (the tensor fascia lata passes over two joints--the knee joint *and* the hip joint. I really should call it the knee and hip joint destroyer.)

Start by attempting to ripple the skin of this area, by bringing your thumb toward your fingers. Notice how thick the skin is, and how it resists your attempts to ripple it. In a minute or two you will very likely begin experiencing a considerable amount of pain--a lot of hidden pain has been stored up in those tissues. The tensor fascia lata is a knee stabilizer. Every time you take a step it absorbs some stress and develops more hidden pain. I know when I treated my tensor fascia lata several years ago, I was *astonished* by the large amount of pain my explorations revealed.

I think you will find that the skin of the tensor fascia lata is bonded to deeper tissues. Dysfunctioning tissue systems have a capability of getting "glued" or bonded to one another. Skin gets bonded to fascia, fascia gets bonded to muscles. Even ligaments can get bonded to other tissues. These bonds will break up and disappear with gentle explorations.

Now try single finger sweeps along the entire tensor fascia lata, from hip to beyond the knee joint--to get an idea of its dimensions. Notice that it's wide, up at the hip, and narrows as it approaches the knee. Refer to the drawing on p. 146.

Go back to skin ripplings. Then place your hand over the tensor fascia lata, so your palm is resting on it, with your thumb on one side and your fingers on the other. Gently move the tensor fascia lata, side to side-- from hip down to its attachment beyond the knee. This gentle exploring movement will help break the bonds mentioned above.

You have now explored/treated the tissues primarily responsible for causing knee pain. With continued self-treatments, your tissues will become healthier and healthier--until, as mentioned above--your knee pain will be a thing of the past.

By the way, if your doctor has been talking about replacing your knee with a mechanical one, ask him/her to read this book.

An important word of caution! Whenever treating your leg, particularly your calf, check first to see if it seems unusually warm, red or swollen. If so, do not treat and see your doctor immediately. This could be a sign of a serious health condition known as DVT (deep vein thrombosis) that could be life-threatening. Indeed, even if these warning signs are absent, I strongly suggest that readers visit their doctors before treating their legs to rule out any possibility of having this condition.

Logger's Hand

Hands can be abused by all sorts of trauma. As a case in point, I present the following.

Case History

I coined the term "logger's hand" to describe a patient I treated a few years ago. The gentleman was in his mid-forties and had been a logger since his mid-teens. For thirty years, he had worked in all extremes of weather and had received numerous injuries, including fractures to his hands and arms. He had pulled heavy log chains with his bare hands, had used all kinds of heavy equipment that injured his hands, and had generally abused his hands to an extent I have not observed before or since.

The result was a pair of hands that were almost completely non-functional. He was unable to work as a logger because he could not hold or use a chain saw or any other logging equipment. Most sadly, he had a three-year-old, and he told me, with tears in his eyes, that he was so helpless he could not even button the child's clothing. He was reluctant to try my treatments but came because a friend who knew of my work had insisted.

His hands and fingers were thick, stiff, and painful. He could bend his fingers only very slightly. He held his hands with his fingers outstretched. The tissues of the rest of his upper extremities were also affected, but not nearly so much as his hands.

At the beginning of the first visit, he held out his hands and said, "There ain't no way that anybody can help these-here hands." After the first treatment was over, however, he had to admit that his fingers did seem to be a "little looser," and his hands did feel a "little better."

We continued treatment twice a week for eight weeks. At the end of this time, he had regained full use of his hands, although some mid-palm tightness remained. He had resumed full-time work as a logger and was able to button his child's clothing. He was discharged, happy and pleased.

The Schatz Technique™ Instructions

For suggestions for *The Schatz Technique™* treatment, refer to "Carpal Tunnel Syndrome."

Migraine and Muscle

Contraction/Tension Headaches

The current medical system contends there are primarily two kinds of head pain, which they name migraine and muscle contraction headaches. Doctors admit they do not know what causes migraines but think they are associated somehow with vascular dysfunction of a vague and ill-defined nature. They consider migraines to be incurable.

Doctors think muscle contraction headache, sometimes called tension headache, is caused by contracted or tense muscles. This is getting a little closer to the truth, but their analysis is so simplistic that any treatment value is lost. The current medical system considers migraine and "muscle contraction" headaches to be unrelated. Unable to treat the cause, doctors attempt to "manage" the pain of all headaches with drugs.

Several years ago, I became aware of the relationship of head pain to soft tissue dysfunction. When I treated patients for upper back problems, I noted that they frequently stated they also suffered from headaches. Some had been diagnosed as having migraine headaches, others as having muscle contraction headaches. The interesting thing was that both types of headaches became milder and less frequent as the tight and contracted tissues of their backs softened and became pain-free.

As I gained experience, I refined my ability to identify and treat the tissues that cause headaches. I now know it is extremely important to examine the scalp, face, neck, and upper chest, as well as the back, for tight, contracted, and fibrotic areas. When these are identified and palpated, a headache will frequently be elicited, which *confirms* the relationship of soft tissue dysfunction and the headache symptom.

I now know it is extremely important to examine the scalp, face, neck, and upper chest, as well as the back, for tight, contracted, and fibrotic areas. When these are found and palpated, a headache will frequently be elicited, which confirms the relationship of soft tissue dysfunction and the headache symptom.

Another frequent response to this procedure is this: "Oh, that's just where I get my headache!"

It is necessary to treat, reverse, and normalize all dysfunctioning tissues found to contribute to your headache symptoms for you to become free of pain and stay free of pain.

Scalp. Your scalp is not just a piece of skin stretched over the skull to provide a foundation for hair to grow out of. It contains an extensive network of stress-receiving, stress-storing, and stress-triggering tissues. When these become tight, contracted, and fibrotic, they send out alarm signals of pain that are called migraine and muscle contraction headaches.

Face. Tissues of your face should be soft, supple, and free of pain. Tissues underlying the skin at the nasal sinuses should not be hard, thick, or painful, nor should the tissues around your eyes. When skin under the jaw line is gently moved between the thumb and fingers, it should not feel lumpy or painful. These are all signs of soft tissue dysfunction that likely contribute to your headache.

Tissues of the face receive, absorb, and store messages of internal and external stress. Creases form with fibrotic tissue underlying each crease. The greater the accumulation of stress, the thicker the underlying layer of fibrotic tissue, and the deeper the crease. As this process continues year after year, more and more tissue dysfunction develops, and higher levels of hidden pain are stored away.

The face is the primary area of the body that expresses our emotions. In order to express emotions, its tissues have to be strong receivers of emotional messages, many of which are stressful in nature. Look at photographs of Abraham Lincoln taken at different times as the Civil War progressed. You can see how the tissues of his face changed, how they became tight, contracted, and fibrotic.

Constantly bombarded by these messages, the tissues of the face become part of a stress loop, later sending stress messages back out to the body. So one might say that the individual causes his face to become stressed. On the other hand, the face causes the individual to become stressed.

Your face should be treated, not only to improve your appearance and to normalize painful areas, but also to reduce the stress signals that are being sent out so you can become fully healthy again. Just as with other areas of your body, the tissues of your face will respond to proper treatment by becoming soft and supple. You will be astonished how relaxed and stress-free you become after the tissues of your face are properly treated and released, and your headaches go away.

Neck: The tissues of your neck should be soft and supple. The two bands of muscles at the front of the neck (sternocleidomastoids) and their associated tissues should not be hard or painful to examination, particularly at their upper ends where they attach behind the ears. All the tissues of the neck (front, sides, and back) should be carefully examined for areas of dysfunction. They are frequently headache generators and must be normalized if pain-free health is to be achieved.

Back: The tissues of your back, particularly the upper back, are important contributors of head pain. The trapezius muscle is almost always involved. Its job is to hold your head upright; therefore, it is in a state of constant tension whenever you sit, stand, or walk about. The only time it has to rest is when you lie down. This constant tension causes the muscle to become extremely tight, contracted, and fibrotic (i.e., dysfunctional). The signals of distress it sends out adds to your headache.

Chest: The pectoral muscles and their associated tissues, located at your chest, can be contributors of head pain. They also have to be examined and if found to be dysfunctional, must be treated, if freedom from headaches is to be achieved.

Case History 1

I was speaking with a young neurology resident at a teaching hospital. In the course of our conversation, I mentioned that I treated migraine patients. I told her of some of my experiences and explained my treatment rationale. She became very interested and said that she and her associates would keep me busy treating migraine patients, as there was a long list of them in her department that were suffering severe pain and not being helped.

The resident said that just that morning she had examined a twenty-six-year-old woman who had suffered migraines for nine years. She experienced severe migraines daily, and every few days was so incapacitated by a particularly excruciating migraine that she had to go to an emergency room for injections of pain medication. The woman told her that these episodes of increased pain, accompanied by nausea and vomiting, were nightmarish.

The patient had just returned from an extensive workup at a new multimillion-dollar headache center, where she was told that nothing more could be done to reduce the severity or frequency of her migraines.

The neurology resident said she would immediately refer this woman for treatment and that numerous referrals from the doctors in her unit would soon follow. I told her to please limit the referrals to not more than ten. This would allow me the time necessary to treat each one on a quality basis.

The young woman did call, and we started treatment the next day. When I examined her, I found the tissues of her scalp, neck, upper back and chest to be severely contracted. Particularly affected were the tissues of her scalp and neck. Her scalp was drawn tight as a drum and was intensely painful to the lightest touch.

I treated her daily in two-hour sessions. The first treatments were stormy, because even lightly touching the affected areas elicited a headache. But she continued to return for further treatment for two reasons: one, the very fact that touching the tight, contracted tissue caused a headache demonstrated that the tight, contracted tissue was the underlying cause of her headaches; and two, after each treatment she felt her body becoming looser.

After the first few treatments, the reactions became milder, and she noticed that between treatments her headaches were less severe and less frequent. After three weeks, she reported that she had gone two days without a headache. She considered this to be a miracle.

I continued to treat her daily for three months. During this time, her tissues progressively softened, and, although there were days when she still experienced a severe headache, their intensity and frequency diminished. She no longer required emergency-room visits.

The next two months brought continued improvement. Most days were completely headache-free. Occasionally, she experienced a mild headache. Her quality of life had dramatically improved.

I sent reports to the neurology department and to the resident who had made the referral, describing how the patient was improving, but I received no reply from them. Nor did I receive any more referrals of the "many migraine patients that were not being helped."

The doctors could see her dramatic improvement, and could hear her comments describing her improvement, when she reported for rechecks to their department. Yet, to my puzzlement, no more migraine sufferers were referred to me. One day, as I was chatting with my patient, I mentioned my puzzlement to her.

"How naive you are, Bernard. Don't you understand what happened? When the resident reported to her chief that she had referred me to you, she was probably reprimanded and told, 'We do the migraine patients here, we do not refer them out.'"

I would have wanted to continue to treat this patient to get her completely free of pain, but she moved away from the area. I received a letter from her two years later saying that she was continuing to do well with no return of prior symptoms. It is unfortunate that this young woman had to endure those nine nightmarish years when appropriate treatment early on could probably have prevented *any* headaches from developing.

Case History 2

A young woman was referred to me because of excruciating headaches that had been occurring daily for over a year. The headaches started at the back of her head, continued over her scalp, and ended in agonizing pain behind her eyes. Her doctor had diagnosed them as muscle contraction headaches. She described the pain as "terrible" and "unbearable." The pain medications and muscle relaxants her doctor had given her had not helped, and she told me she was ready for God to take her.

When I examined her, I found that the tissues of her upper back, neck, and scalp were severely contracted, and the overlying skin was drawn tight and adherent to the underlying tissues. All these tissues were extremely tender to mild examination. She tolerated only the mildest of treatment for the first week. Gradually, as her tissues loosened and softened, she tolerated more treatment, and her headaches lessened in intensity and frequency.

At the end of a month, she no longer experienced any headaches. I continued treatment at decreasing frequency for two more months, until I could no longer feel any tight or contracted tissues.

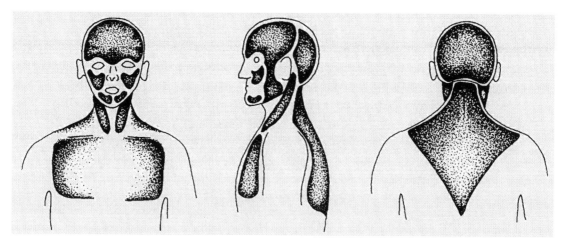

Primary areas of contracted tissues that cause headaches

Here was a case that doctors had called a "muscle contraction" headache, but that was a misdiagnosis. Her skin, muscles, and fascia were tight, thick, and fibrotic. The muscles were not contracted in the common sense, and there is no pain medication or muscle relaxant in the world that could have reversed and normalized this woman's problem.

The Schatz Technique™ **Instructions**

Important areas to be treated include (1) scalp, (2) face, (3) neck, (4) upper back, and (5) chest.

Other body areas may be affected, but the above are almost always involved. Start your treatment lying face up and support your head comfortably, with as many pillows as needed.

Treating your scalp. Start your headache treatment at the scalp. The scalp is the one and only area where lotion should not be used. I tried it once. Trust me, it doesn't work. Your hair itself will act as a sort of "lubricant." However, if part of your scalp is hair deficient, you can use lotion there.

Take your time and get acquainted with your scalp. Slip one hand behind your head so the palm supports the back of your head. This will free your thumb and fingers to explore and treat. Use your fingertips, all of them at the same time, to make exploratory circles. Start with small circles. Enlarge the circles. Try slow circles, then faster ones. Try back-and-forths with all your fingers. Now use your forefinger as the primary probe. As you continue with your scalp (and other tissue area) explorations, try the different finger configurations described in the glossary. Refer to it from time to time for *The Schatz Technique™* suggestions; try variations of pressure. Press firmly. Press lightly.

Alternate your right and left examining hands frequently so they do not get fatigued. As you gently explore the various areas of your scalp, move the supporting palm accordingly: from the back of your head, to the right side, left side, and to the front.

The purpose of all this is to find and soften tight, painful areas. Scalp dysfunction can take various forms. Have your fingers look for very small, hard, painful, fibrotic knots. Move your fingers carefully, or you may miss some. When you find one, stay with it. If it is very painful, lighten your touch, but stay with it. Try very small back-and-forths, circles, or stationary probes on that painful, hard knot. You will likely feel the pain ease and disappear. If you then move off the area, you won't be able to find the knot again. *It will no longer be there.*

Something may happen when you press on that knot: It may trigger a headache. It seems ironic, to try to help yourself and then cause a headache. It's as if you're pressing a headache button. The only way you can soften that button and make it go away, so it will eventually cease causing headaches, is to gently touch and soothe it.

It would have been far better if this had been properly treated years earlier, before things became so severe. But unfortunately this was not done, and you now have no choice but to deal with your present reality. You must work on that knot until it goes away, so lighten your touch to the weight of a feather. It may be that it is so established that it will not soften in one treatment; it may take several treatments to soften and normalize it. If so, that is what you will have to do. Be assured that persistence and coaxing will pay off.

Something else may happen when you press on that knot. You may, for example, feel pain generated at a distant point, perhaps your shoulder or chest. This is one of those TCF loops (tight, contracted, fibrotic) mentioned earlier in this book. When this happens, I suggest that you also work on the shoulder or chest. Chances are you will then feel pain generated back up to your scalp. Both areas have to be normalized.

Another form of scalp dysfunction is a band of tight, contracted tissue. A pair can usually be found running from the forehead backward to where the skull starts curving down, bordering the area where men frequently are bald. These can be stubborn and resistant to softening. Double-finger back-and-forths are helpful here. Be patient and persistent. More than one session will probably be required.

Yet another configuration of dysfunction is a broad area of tight tissue just above and behind each ear, near where the sternocleidomastoid muscle attaches. These can be extremely tender and painful. Try gentle circles, back-and-forths, and stationary presses. It is important to resolve these areas. (Refer to the section "Ear Pain" for detailed instructions.)

Work back and to the sides, toward your temples. You undoubtedly will find severely thickened and tender tissue there–this is where the temporomandibular muscle attaches, an important area.

When you go back as far as you can before you run into the pillows supporting your head, turn your head to one side so you can reach the back of your scalp. This will get you to your occipital area, where your posterior neck muscles attach. This area is of extreme importance. Treat it carefully and thoroughly with firm (but gentle) thumb and finger circles. Then turn to the other side and treat the remaining area of scalp tissue.

When all areas have been treated, go back and give a nice, light "once-over" to tie everything together. Use all fingers of both hands in broad circular sweeps. When you do this, think of getting the circulation going all through your scalp.

You can easily have spent two hours in your scalp exploration and treatment. I hope you found it interesting, and that you now realize your scalp is an area of great complexity and importance.

Treating your face. After you treat your scalp, I suggest you move down to your face. Now you will need lotion and a cup of warm water. The forehead is a good place to start. Apply a small amount of lotion there. Place the thumb of your examining hand under your cheekbone. That will give you leverage and control when your fingers are placed on your forehead. Begin by examining some skin creases. Try small circles on a crease; be gentle. Then try stationary and side-to-side presses. Do you feel pain deep in the crease? Does it trigger pain to another area of your face? Up to your scalp? Behind an eye? Is it associated with your headaches?

Move along the entire length of the crease. Take your time. If the lotion dries out, apply a bit more, or perhaps a drop or two of water. If you like the feel of friction when you work on the crease, apply additional lotion later. Thoroughly explore the crease, then move on to another crease.

Perhaps you are curious because your fingers found an area of hardened skin, so gently explore that area of skin. Does it become painful after a moment or two of gentle examination? Does it trigger pain elsewhere? Is it associated with your headaches? Gently squeeze that area of skin. Can you ripple it? Is it adherent to the tissues underneath? Does it become more painful as you work with it? Does it begin to soften as you work with it? Does the pain lessen?

Don't forget to change hands from time to time so they don't get tired.

Try some large sweeps across your entire forehead. Sweep across all your forehead creases. Try some large back-and-forths with all your fingers. Whenever you find something interesting (painful, hard, adherent, thick), pause and gently work on it. Now concentrate on the area just above your eyebrows. Try a variety of movements. Move down to the eyebrows proper.

Don't rush; always take your time. Go wherever your fingers lead you. Learn to trust your fingers.

Explore your entire forehead, up to your scalp line and down to the bridge of your nose. The tissue at the bridge of your nose can be an important component of headache production. Try pincering it firmly with a static hold. Do you feel pain developing? Does it radiate to your eyes? To your head? Is it associated with your headaches?

Move out to the sides of your forehead, to your temples. You will be forgiven if you intrude back onto your scalp, where your temporomandibular muscle attaches, for another going-over there.

Now place a forefinger at each depression just behind the ridge at the outer edge of your eyes. Move your forefingers in small, firm circles. Any pain there? If you find some (you likely will), follow it. Does it go back up to your forehead? Any association with your headaches? Do you find thick, contracted tissues? Will these tissues need further treatment?

Place some lotion on your face on either side of your nose (the sort of triangle between your nose and your cheekbones). Explore these areas carefully with back-and-forths and circles. Do they feel thickened and tight? Is one side thicker than the other? Any pain there? Any association with your headache? When you press there, is a headache generated?

These are your sinus areas. It is very likely they will need continued care before they become softened, normalized, and healthy. (Refer to the sections titled "Sinus Headache" and "Sinus Pain" for more detailed instructions.)

Work down the tissues overlying your jaws. It is likely these tissues are dysfunctional and important pain generators. Brace your thumb on the underside of your jaw. This will give your exploring fingers leverage and control. Thoroughly investigate and treat these tissues with the variety of techniques you are now getting familiar with.

Check the tissues that are closely attached to your jawbone. Follow its entire length. Look for hard, wire like, adherent formations toward the front of the jaw. Run your thumb back and forth. Any pain in these? (Refer to "TMJ Pain" for detailed instructions on treating jaw tissues.)

You have now explored and treated your face and scalp. Did you find areas that are associated with your headache? I would be surprised if you didn't. Are you surprised at what you found? Were your explorations interesting? Do you feel you know more about your body? Your headaches?

You are now ready to proceed with your headache treatment.

Treating your neck and upper back. Tissues of your neck are a continuation of tissues of your trunk. I am speaking of the major neck muscles: the pair of sternocleidomastoids in the front, and the trapezius in the back. It is important to treat these muscles thoroughly, particularly where they attach to the back of the head.

The sternocleidomastoids are the two long, narrow muscles that begin at the upper chest, run up the front of your neck, and attach just behind your ears. The trapezius is the broad, thick muscle of your upper back; it attaches to the occipital area at the back of your head (see diagram p. 50). It is the muscle that gets increasingly tight and painful as the day progresses.

I suggest you treat your sternocleidomastoids first. (Please note that whenever muscles are mentioned, their associated skin and fascia must also be treated.)

Lie face up, with your head on extra pillows, so it is tilted forward. This will put some slack in your sternocleidomastoids and make it easier for you to work on them. Start at the middle of either the right or left muscle. Let us say you start with the one on your right.

167

Grasp it between your thumb and the knuckle of your forefinger and gently roll it back and forth. This will likely elicit some level of discomfort, so be very gentle. Do this for a few seconds, then move downward toward your trunk. Continue treating until you reach the part that is attached to your collarbone (that's the cleido part of sternocleidomastoid). Work the collarbone attachment with circles, back-and-forths, and double-finger nudges. You will likely find painful tissue there.

Continue along your collarbone toward the center of your chest, toward your sternum (the sterno part of the name). Work this area carefully, again with circles, back-and-forths, and double finger nudges.

Turn your head to the right so you are looking toward your right shoulder. This will slacken the muscle where it attaches to the bump behind the ear, the mastoid process, an important headache area. Go back to the middle of the muscle and work up to where it is firmly attached to your head, where you can't move it anymore. Probe this area thoroughly with your fore and middle fingers held together. Feel free to go back up into your scalp if interesting things draw you there. Use your thumb to explore and treat. I feel certain you will find significant pain areas here. Do you?

When you have explored this sternocleidomastoid thoroughly, treat the other one in a similar manner. Don't forget to turn your head to the left when you work on its mastoid attachment.

You will now treat your trapezius. It may not seem feasible to treat tissues at the back of your neck and down between the upper part of your shoulders, but it can be done. I know, because I have treated myself in these areas.

Arrange the pillows so your head is tilted backward, giving the muscle some slack. Remember, the trapezius is responsible for keeping your head upright throughout the day. It works continuously, never relaxing, and is truly a stressed and dysfunctional muscle. Accordingly, it underlies many pain problems, including headaches. Persistence and patience are required to normalize it.

The palm of your examining hand is behind your head. Place your fingers on one side of the attachment of the trapezius, and your thumb on the other. Use your thumb to make small, firm circles where the muscle attaches. This may lead you back into the scalp.

Continue making firm circles; do the same with the fingers. Thoroughly examine the attachment area. Follow painful, thick tissues, even if this leads you away from the trapezius.

After you explore these, make your way back to the attachment. Work slowly. Undoubtedly, you will find an abundance of things to work on. Change hands from time to time to avoid fatigue. Gently pincer the muscle below the attachment between your thumb and forefinger. Coax it with push-pulls, then little circles. Try gentle kneading movements. Work down two or three inches, to where the muscle begins to widen. Now, with your right hand, reach around your front toward the back of your left shoulder. You will rest your palm on your collarbone, allowing your thumb and fingers free to explore the trapezius.

Because you are lying on your back, your trapezius will be as relaxed as possible. Press upward into the muscle with all your fingers held close together. Use soothing circles. Do you get the feeling that your careworn trapezius is saying, "Ah, relief at last"? No doubt you will find tight, contracted, and fibrotic areas throughout. Explore and soothe. Use your thumb to make circles into the muscle. Pincer it between thumb and fingers and perform push-pulls. Don't forget to treat the skin overlying your trapezius.

Work down to your shoulder blade. I'll wager you will find pain there. Treat this area thoroughly. Treat the portion of the trapezius that attaches to your spinal column; circle each vertebrae; work down as far as you can reach. Don't rush; let your tissues enjoy their long-neglected bliss. When you have done this to your tissues' satisfaction, use your left hand to treat your right trapezius. Although your trapezius will require patient and persistent treatment, your efforts will be rewarded when it no longer contributes to your headaches.

Treating your chest. Apply some lotion to the inner side of your shoulder at the level of your collarbone. Use small single and multiple finger circles and move horizontally, just under your collarbone, toward the center of your chest to the sternum.

Enlarge the circles until they sweep the area enclosed by an imaginary line from the shoulder joint to the top of the sternum, down the sternum, out to the rib cage, then back up to the shoulder joint. This will form a rectangle I call the chest rectangle.

Explore and treat the tissues attached to the collarbone, using all your fingers to sweep horizontally, then try small multiple finger circles for the same tissues. Treat the skin with thumb ripples. When you come to where the sternocleidomastoids are attached, feel free to re-explore those muscles and their associated tissues.

Carefully explore down the sternum using multiple-finger circles and back and forth strokes. When you come to the bottom of the sternum, continue the multiple-finger circles out to where you can feel your ribs.

Continue upward toward the original starting point of the shoulder joint. The tissue along this rim of the chest rectangle is the outer edge of the pectoral muscle. When treating this area of the right pectoral, use your left hand. Place the palm of your hand on your chest. Position your thumb on the front of the edge of the muscle with your fingers curled around and behind it.

Every cubic centimeter of dysfunctional tissue has to be treated and normalized if full health is to be attained. Keep at it. It takes work and dedication. But it will be worth all the effort when your headaches are gone and your body feels wonderful again.

Pincer the muscle between thumb and fingers. Use your index finger to perform circles upward into the muscle.

Examine and treat in this manner along the entire edge of the muscle. When you reach the shoulder joint, bring your fingers to the front and use multiple-finger circles and thumb sweeps. Continue with single and double finger movements. Be very gentle here, because it is an area that can contain severe hidden pain. Use plenty of lotion diluted with water so your fingers and thumb can slip easily over your skin. You may be surprised how much pain you find here, so go slowly. You may be further surprised that in just a few days it is likely you will no longer find any pain there; the area will be healthy. Treat the opposite side in a similar manner.

You now have finished treating the tissues that are the primary headache generators. Did you notice how quickly the time went? Every cubic centimeter of dysfunctional tissue has to be treated and normalized if full health is to be attained. Keep at it. It takes work and dedication. But it will be worth all the effort when your headaches are gone and your body feels wonderful again.

Muscle Weakness

When muscles become infiltrated with fibrotic tissue, they lose their elasticity and ability to perform efficiently. They become weak. Exercise does not improve this kind of weakness, even though doctors prescribe it for this condition. Many patients who complain of increasing weakness of their arms, hands, and fingers are put on exercise programs by their doctors in a misguided attempt. Dysfunctional tissues need to be healed before an exercise program is begun.

Patients are recycled year after year through "strengthening" programs, only to grow weaker. These individuals come to me because of the severe pain they are experiencing. I learn of their weakness when I examine them. The interesting thing is when I treat and reverse the tight, fibrotic tissue that causes their pain, their strength increases, frequently quite dramatically, at the very first treatment. It is a wonderful experience to have someone come for a treatment experiencing severe pain and weakness, and have them leave with little or no pain and normal, or normal strength.

In these cases, their muscles were weaker because the muscle fibers were bound by tight, fibrotic tissue. This was near the same tight, fibrotic tissue that was pressing on pain receptors and causing the pain that brought them to me. When I softened and released the fibrotic tissue, their muscles were able to function normally, and their strength returned. The exercise programs they were on only stimulated the production of additional fibrotic tissue.

Case History

A man in his mid-sixties was referred because of severely painful hands. His problem, diagnosed as arthritis, had progressed over a four-year period. In addition to the pain, his hands had become increasingly weak. His doctor sent him to the rehabilitation department of a nearby teaching hospital, where he participated in several exercise programs. However, the exercises had not increased or even maintained his strength. When I saw him, he could barely hold a set of keys; his grip was so weak he was unable to shake my hand.

When I examined him, I noted that the tissues of both hands and forearms were tight and contracted. His tissues responded rapidly, and at the end of the two-hour treatment he happily reported that he had very little pain. I asked if he could now shake my hand, and he did so with a firm grip. He was delighted by his increased strength and decreased pain.

The Schatz Technique™ **Instructions**

If your hands and arms are weak and painful, refer to "Carpal Tunnel Syndrome." Other areas likely to be weakened by soft tissue dysfunction are the hips and knees. Refer to those sections for treatment suggestions.

Musician's Pain

Musicians stress their bodies by placing them in uncomfortable positions for long hours of practice year after year. Imperceptively at first many find their techniques compromised by the development of tight, contracted tissues. For some, their careers end because of incapacitating pain and dysfunction.

Musicians, who devote years of their lives to aesthetic study, receive the same inappropriate treatment for their pain as the rest of the population. The treatment the current medical system doles out to their musician patients includes: exercise, rest, pain medication, cortisone injections, stretching, surgery, heat, splinting and psychiatric care. These remedies however have no effect in normalizing the extensive soft tissue dysfunction that takes place in the bodies of musicians.

A few years ago, I attended a symposium titled "Performing Arts Medicine: Issues in Diagnosis and Management." Several prestigious doctors were mentioned as presenters, among whom was Dr. A, with an international reputation as a specialist in musicians' problems. Also mentioned as a presenter was Dr. B, a physician with considerable experience in the care of musicians and performing artists.

On the first day of the symposium, I introduced myself to Dr. B as I was interested in what he thought of my approach to treating soft tissue dysfunction in musicians. But Dr. B showed no interest in my approach or my findings. After a moment or two he walked off, ending our conversation.

The last session of the symposium was a session cochaired by Dr. A and Dr. B. Following a few prefatory remarks, the session was open to audience participation. Immediately, a woman rose and tearfully related that she had been a woodwind soloist, but over a ten-year period had developed severe and progressive pain and tightness in her upper back and both arms. Eventually the pain and tightness had become so severe she gave up her musical career. At this point, she broke down completely, and a minute or two passed before she then composed herself.

She continued: after the ending of her career as a soloist, she began teaching, but this too was becoming increasingly difficult because of excruciating pain. Hearing of the symposium she was attending to ask the doctors what they could do to help her.

Well, here it comes. Now I will hear what these eminent, doctors do to treat musicians. I had my thoughts as to how I would treat this woman–softening and normalizing the tight, contracted, fibrotic tissue that undoubtedly was the cause of her pain and dysfunction.

To my astonishment Dr. A told this suffering musician that nothing could be done for her. Her case was much too advanced. Had she come to them years earlier, maybe something could have been done; Dr. B agreed.

The woman thanked them, murmuring that was what she thought they would say but had come just in case. She sat down sobbing. This was unfortunate. There was a great deal that could be done for this woman as I had successfully treated many people who had considerably worse symptoms than she described.

I was in a dilemma. Should I stand and say I thought I could help her? Based on my extensive experience as exemplified by the brief encounter with Dr. B at the coffee break, I decided against it. I didn't want to be disruptive. I determined instead to go over to her after the session, give her my card, and tell her that I could offer her at least a glimmer of hope.

Next, a young man stood and stated he was a guitarist and that over the past two years was gradually developing pain and tightness in his arms and hands. He could still play well, but his technique was beginning to be affected. He asked the doctors for their help.

Now, I would learn the doctors' approach to treating a musician! Here was a musician with early signs of pain and dysfunction. I leaned forward in my chair and eagerly awaited their remarks.

Dr. A told this musician the same thing he told the previous one: his case was too advanced. If he had come earlier, maybe something could have been done, but now it was too late. Dr. B agreed.

This was too much! This musician had early, *easily* treatable dysfunction. I could picture the condition of the tissues of his arms and hands and how they would respond to care. I couldn't believe the doctors had told him that nothing could be done. I determined to also speak with him after the session ended.

At the close of the session, I did approach both musicians. I told them I could offer help. I handed each a card and asked them to call me. Neither did.

For years, I have puzzled over the response of the doctors to the entreaties of these two suffering musicians. Why did the doctors not suggest appropriate treatment? The answer came: the doctors didn't treat musicians; they attempted to managed them, just as the symposium said: "Performing Arts Medicine: Issues in Diagnosis and *Management*."

Case History 1

A young woman called one day. She had been a harpsichordist with a promising career, but two years earlier, while preparing for an important concert, her hands and arms became painfully tight, and she found that she was unable to play at all. She had been to several doctors, but nothing could be done for her. She had reluctantly come to the realization that she would never play again.

She had recently heard of me from a musician friend I had helped and had obtained a referral allowing me to treat. She lived several hours away and could only come on weekends. When she arrived for her first treatment, I learned that for several weeks prior to her final concert she had been under severe emotional strain due to serious illness in her family. That, and the emotional and physical stress of strenuous rehearsals, had put the final touches on a condition that had most likely been developing over time.

When I examined her, I found the tissues of her neck, back, shoulders, forearms, wrists, and fingers were tight, contracted, and painful when lightly palpated. The tissues of her hands and fingers were thick and she could only move her fingers slowly, with great pain.

I treated her for five weekends, in four-to-five hour sessions. At the end of this time, the affected tissues had softened appreciably and she could move her fingers with very little pain. She started to play again. She was delighted. I wanted to continue treating until her body was completely normalized, but she was pleased that she could play again. Since she no longer had aspirations of resuming a serious career, she was satisfied with her level of recovery, and treatments were discontinued.

Case History 2

A flutist who contacted me said that twenty years earlier she had injured the distal joint (the end joint) of her little finger. The joint had remained stiff over the years and in the past couple of years had stiffened even more. The area around the joint was becoming increasingly painful, and her technique was affected.

She had heard of my work from another musician and wondered if I could help her. In examination I found fibrotic development around her affected joint, which prevented it from moving properly. The limited area of tissue dysfunction responded very rapidly to treatment, and she was completely pain and symptom free in three sessions and needed no further treatment.

Case History 3

A young female pre-med student, was experiencing severe pain in her left (dominant) arm, such that it was seriously affecting her note-taking. She heard of my work and called to make an appointment. I told her I needed a doctor's referral in order to treat her. When she arrived for her first treatment, I learned she had been a serious student of the violin; however, after years of long hours of practice, her body and left arm had gradually become so painful that four years earlier she had stopped playing altogether.

Now as a pre-med student note taking had caused the old pain to flare up with a vengeance. She was greatly concerned that the same pain that had ended her career as a violinist was now ending her opportunity of becoming a doctor.

Upon examining her, I found contracted and painful tissue of her neck, left pectoral area, shoulder girdle, and down through her left arm and into her hand and fingers. Her pain rapidly reduced within two weeks, allowing her to resume note-taking, but two months of treatment was necessary to normalize the severely contracted tissue of her pectoral, cervical, and shoulder girdle areas and avoid future problems.

At discharge, she was completely pain and symptom free. Her dysfunctioning tissues had been normalized.

The Schatz Technique™ Instructions

Your problem may be occurring anywhere in your body. Frequently, shoulders, arms, and hands are involved. Refer to "Carpal Tunnel Syndrome" for treatment suggestions. The neck, back, and hips are also likely areas of tissue dysfunction and pain. Refer to those sections for treatment techniques.

Neck Pain

Soft tissue dysfunction is frequently the underlying cause of neck pain. The pain can be caused by tissues directly associated with the neck or tissues that lie far from it.

Case History

I received a call from a twenty-eight-year-old woman who said she had been suffering excruciating neck pain for two years. The pain was continuous, with not a moment of relief since it began. She had been treated by five practitioners: three medical doctors, a chiropractor, and a physical therapist. None had been able to help as nothing had shown up on her X-rays or other tests, and her neck pain continued unabated.

She had given up all hope and had resigned herself to a life of pain when someone told her of my work. She asked if I thought I could help her. I suggested she get a doctor's referral that would allow me to examine and treat her, and we would then see what might be done.

When she came in for treatment, I learned she had been extremely busy with a computer project for three years. The only pain of which she was aware was a severe pain on the right side of her neck. Her neck area was so painful to the touch that she could not tolerate even the lightest touch. When I applied lotion and gently examined the tissues of her right shoulder, arm, forearm, hand, and fingers, she was astonished at the severity of hidden pain that was revealed in those areas. She had not been aware of any pain before my gentle explorations.

Equally astonishing to her was the fact that when I touched those areas her neck pain became even more severe. There was also one small spot in the web of her thumb that seemed particularly connected to her neck pain.

Her neck was so tender that at first she could not tolerate even the lightest touch there. When I applied lotion and gently examined the tissues of her right shoulder, arm, forearm, hand, and fingers, she was astonished at the severity of hidden pain that was revealed in those areas. There was also one small spot in the web of her thumb that seemed particularly connected to her neck pain.

When I gently pressed it, her neck pain became unbearable. She was also surprised when I pointed out how tight and thick the muscles attached to her elbow were, as well as the tissues of her hand, fingers and thumb. Dysfunctioning tissue was also found in her upper and mid-back, and down her left upper extremity, although not as severe as her right side.

After two hours of treatment, I noted that the tissues of her neck, back, and right upper extremity had softened, and she reported that her pain was almost gone and her body felt looser and lighter.

She continued to respond rapidly and after only four more treatments was discharged completely free of pain. I sent reports of her progress to her primary physician, the one who had sent her to those other practitioners, but did not receive a reply or query as to what I had done to successfully treat this previously "unhelpable" patient who had been prepared to live the rest of her life in excruciating pain.

The Schatz Technique™ **Instructions**

If your neck pain is caused by dysfunctioning soft tissue (organic or structural causation being ruled out), then all areas that might be contributing to the pain must be examined and normalized.

Tissue areas most likely to cause neck pain include

1. **the head**
2. **the neck itself**
3. **the upper back**
4. **the upper extremities.**

For *The Schatz Technique*™ treatment instructions for the head, neck, and upper back refer to "Migraine and Muscle Contraction Headaches." For instructions that normalize the tissues of the upper extremities, refer to "Carpal Tunnel Syndrome."

Peripheral Vascular Disease

As a physical therapist, I have been involved with the care of ulcers referred to as "wound care" and caused by what doctors call peripheral vascular disease. My direct experience with this problem goes back almost half a century.

Not once in all these years have I seen a doctor carefully examine the tissues of a patient suffering from peripheral vascular disease. The reader may find it difficult to believe that not one doctor responded to my entreaty to even touch those tissues; nevertheless, this is so.

A question I have asked doctors repeatedly over the years is, "What is peripheral vascular disease?" There is usually some hesitation before an answer is given, which usually runs along the line of: "Peripheral vascular disease is a problem caused by fatty deposits that narrow blood vessels." I then ask, "How do you examine a patient suffering peripheral vascular disease?" The response is invariably the same: "I check the pressure at various levels of the limb."

"Peripheral vascular disease" as a diagnostic category is in fact a vague and imprecise term. I contend the problem may well occur when blood vessels are squeezed by tight, contracted tissues that *surround* them. Doctors are unaware of this possibly because they do not carefully touch their patients.

As years pass and the tissues become progressively tight and contracted, they exert an increasing tourniquet effect on the blood vessels that pass through them, making their job of supplying blood to the tissues of the extremity and returning it to the heart increasingly difficult.

If the problem is arterial, the tissues from the calf down are tight and contracted. Arteries and their subdivisions are squeezed, and the limb, deprived of vital nutrients, becomes desiccated and unhealthy. Ulcers form, and the life of the limb is put at great peril. Some arterial problems are indeed associated with internal fatty deposits, but I suspect that, even with these, contracted tissues surrounding the blood vessels are a contributing factor.

In the case of veins, as they become less able to do their job, the tissues that rely on them to remove fluid become congested and swollen. When doctors discuss venous problems, as in varicose veins, they say the valve leaflets fail. However, they don't understand that the primary cause of peripheral venous failure is dysfunctioning tissue outside the veins. When the tissues of the gluteal area and upper thigh become contracted and squeeze the veins, the venous return becomes difficult. Over time, the back-pressure of trying to return blood through the mass of tight and contracted tissues causes the valves to eventually fail.

The medical community's approach to arterial peripheral vascular disease is to dispense medication or attempt mechanical procedures designed to dilate the squeezed blood vessels. When these attempts fail, a surgical blood vessel bypass may be attempted. This produces a painful, debilitating, and generally unspectacular outcome if the problem that caused the whole thing–tight, contracted, fibrotic tissue–has remained untreated. Venous peripheral vascular disease is currently dealt with ineffectively by applying constricting bandages or stockings to the bloated areas.

The effective treatment for tight, contracted, fibrotic tissues of an extremity is to soften and normalize the dysfunctioning tissues so the blood vessels can efficiently perform their job in a healthy environment. When this is done, the results can be surprisingly beneficial, even in advanced cases. The optimum time to soften and normalize tight tissues of the extremities is early on, before pain, swelling, and ulcers develop. However, proper treatment can be dramatically effective even in late stages.

It is unfortunate that patients suffering the health risk of so called peripheral vascular disease are being subjected to costly, debilitating, ineffective, and painful surgeries (that include amputation) instead of being offered timely and effective treatment.

Case History

A woman in her eighties was referred for treatment. Her daughter had heard of my work and had arranged for the doctor's referral. She told me her mother suffered from peripheral vascular disease of forty years' duration. The pain had worsened as the years had gone by. Medications had not helped reduce the pain or prevent the progress of the problem.

Recently, the pain had become unbearable. She had difficulty taking even a few steps and was unable to get in or out of bed or a chair without help. She was living with her daughter, but because of her growing dysfunction, they were considering a nursing facility.

When I examined her legs, I could see that from mid-calf down to her feet, the skin was a brownish red. When I palpated this area, I found that the tissue was tough and leathery, and it almost had a "wooden" feel; there was no suppleness or softness of the skin and underlying tissue. I could see that, at the juncture where the skin became discolored and hardened, there was an indented line separating it from the tissues above. Farther up from the calves, from her knees to thighs, the tissues were tight and contracted, although not as hardened as the tissue in her calves. All of these areas were tender and painful to even the mildest touch.

I worked on her legs three times a week for two months. At first, she could tolerate only the mildest of treatments. But gradually the tissues softened, and there were indications that the circulation was improving. There was less pain, and the discoloration began to clear; the tissues became pink, at first for just a few seconds, then for a few minutes. Later, as treatment continued, dramatic improvement lasted for several hours between treatments.

By the second month of treatment, she felt improved enough to have the treatments discontinued. At that time, she was experiencing minimal pain, could get in and out of bed and chairs alone, and felt well enough to continue living with her daughter. She told me that she wished she'd had this treatment forty years earlier. It was indeed sad that she hadn't.

The Schatz Technique™ Instructions

I do not recommend that laypersons treat peripheral vascular disease because of the possibility of having an underlying and very serious life-threatening condition called DVT (deep vein thrombosis).

Rotator Cuff Syndrome

The upper extremity moves through a wide range of motion. The shallow socket of the shoulder joint allows this free movement. The job of holding the upper extremity in place is assigned to muscles, fascia and ligaments closely associated with the shoulder joint. These comprise the rotator cuff.

The complex nature of the tissues that allows free movement makes the shoulder vulnerable to injury. Shoulder pathology may well require surgical intervention. And, orthopedic surgeons have developed wonderful skills and perform extremely complicated surgeries that resolve many of these problems.

However, doctors, highly trained as they may be to perform their surgeries, do not have adequate knowledge of soft tissues. They therefore do not understand that pain and physical dysfunction perceived at the shoulder is frequently caused by extensive areas of tissue dysfunction well away from the shoulder. These distant tissues, as well as the rotators themselves, are likely to respond to soft tissue treatment.

Case History 1

I received a call from a woman who said she was suffering from rotator cuff syndrome. She had fallen three months earlier. Doctors had diagnosed the resulting pain and difficulty in moving her shoulder as rotator cuff syndrome. They gave her pain medicine and other medications. In addition, they ordered physical therapy in the form of

186

exercises and stretches; some of the shoulder stretches were applied by pulley. After each physical therapy session, the pain became more severe, and, as the pain worsened, her ability to move her arm became more difficult.

She said she was now unable to use her arm for any activity. When she attempted to move her shoulder, the pain became unbearable. Her doctors suggested surgery, but she was resigned to live with her pain rather than have an operation. A friend told her of my work, and she called to see if I could help. I told her I would need a doctor's referral to examine and treat her. She said she would get one, and we arranged an appointment time.

When she arrived, I noted that she held her arm rigidly to her side. She felt constant pain, and the slightest movement caused the pain to increase. I found that the tissues of her neck, upper back, right chest, and the tissues of her entire right upper extremity from her shoulder down to her hand were spasmed.

Her tissues responded rapidly to treatment. As I worked down from her neck to shoulder to hand, I could feel the tissues softening under my fingers. After two hours, all the treated tissues felt soft and supple. She reported that "the pain had eased." When she sat up, I asked if she could now move her arm. To her astonishment, she moved her arm through a completely normal range of motion without any pain whatever.

I saw her two more times, but there was no return of pain or tissue spasm. She was discharged, delighted and happy. I reported her recovery to the doctor who had signed her referral, but there was no response or inquiry as to what I had done to achieve that non-surgical success.

Case History 2

A physical therapist contacted me with a complaint of pain and tightness of his right shoulder. He had been active years earlier in amateur softball and felt the stress of this activity was responsible for his shoulder problem, which had been diagnosed as rotator cuff syndrome.

The modalities that had been prescribed had not helped, and his motivation and expertise in performing exercises and stretches had not prevented the pain and tightness from worsening, so he decided to try the surgery his doctor recommended. Unfortunately, the pain and tightness continued. That was three years ago.

He knew of my interest in soft tissue dysfunction and wondered if I might be able to help him. He had already obtained a doctor's referral, so we scheduled a treatment session.

When he arrived for treatment, I noted that he had a thirty percent loss of shoulder movement. Examination revealed that the tissues surrounding his right scapula (shoulder blade) were severely contracted and fibrotic. The skin was adherent to the underlying tissues there. I noted the surgical scar, which was also adherent to underlying tissues.

In addition, I found the tissues of his neck, upper back, and down his right upper extremity were severely contracted and fibrotic. The tissues of his left upper extremity were also contracted, but to a lesser degree.

His fibrotic tissues responded slowly to treatment; however, in three months, he was discharged, pain-free and with a full range of motion.

Case History 3

A woman called and said that her daughter, a high school student, was a swimmer who had injured her shoulder the previous season and now was unable to swim competitively. Her doctor had diagnosed the problem as rotator cuff syndrome. She had been given medication, including two cortisone injections, and had gone to a physical therapist for several sessions of exercise and stretches. However, despite these treatments, the pain had grown worse. Her daughter had not been able to compete the previous season and now was very upset because of the prospect of not being able to swim at all in the current season, her final year of high school.

The woman knew of my work because I had helped a classmate of her daughter's, and she wondered if I might also be able to help her child. I told her to get a doctor's referral, and we set up an appointment.

When I applied lotion and examined the tissues of the young swimmer, I did not find considerable soft tissue dysfunction. There was some spasm of the deltoid, the muscle at the top of the shoulder. But, interestingly, there was a small, hard knot about a quarter of an inch in diameter in the center of the muscle. I asked if she knew what that knot was. She said, "Oh, that must have been where they gave me an antibiotic injection a year ago." I asked to see how much shoulder movement she had, and she winced with pain when she attempted to raise her arm.

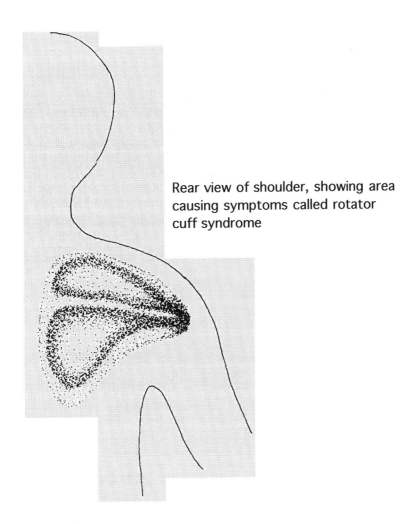

Rear view of shoulder, showing area causing symptoms called rotator cuff syndrome

I worked on her deltoid and its associated tissues for forty minutes and then asked if her arm was any better. She and her mother were surprised and delighted when she moved her arm through a complete range of motion without any pain whatever. Her mother asked if they could have some of that lotion, which she felt must have some sort of magical power to produce such an immediate and dramatic effect. I explained that it was ordinary lotion but gave her some anyway when I saw disbelief on her face.

When they returned for treatment two days later, her daughter was in tears because severe pain had returned. However, I noted the spasm had lessened and the knot was softer. At the end of the session, there was again full movement without pain. With each succeeding treatment, there was less return of pain and spasm. By the sixth session, there was no return of pain or spasm and the knot had disappeared. She was able to swim well the entire season, completely pain and symptom free.

The Schatz Technique™ Instructions

The same tissue areas responsible for symptoms of frozen shoulder are likely the areas that cause rotator cuff syndrome. Treat the tissues of your upper extremity first. Refer to "Carpal Tunnel Syndrome" for *The Schatz Technique*™ instructions. Now treat your chest area. Refer to "Treating your chest" in the section titled "Migraine and Muscle Contraction Headaches." Then treat your upper to lower back tissues. For *The Schatz Technique*™ treatment suggestions for the upper back, refer to "Treating your neck and upper back" in the "Migraine and Muscle Contraction Headaches" section. For the lower back, refer to "Back Pain."

Scars

Scars, whether they have been caused by surgical incision, trauma, or burns, can "hold" pain for years and can be important components of physical dysfunction. The current medical system is apparently unaware of this.

Case History 1

A woman in her fifties was referred because of pain and extreme tightness of her neck and upper back. She said she had had this problem for as long as she could remember, and that it had worsened as time went on. "Pain medication" and "muscle relaxants" had not helped, nor had ultrasound, heat, stretches, or exercises. The referral I received from her doctor called for more of the same, but I called his office and was able to have the referral changed to allow me to treat her properly.

Examination revealed severely thickened and contracted tissues of her middle and upper back, neck, and scalp. These tissues stubbornly resisted treatment, but gradually, after two months of deep work twice a week, her tissues softened, and she felt significant relief.

But not complete relief. We would get her tissues relaxed and softened after a treatment, but by the time she returned for her next treatment, much of the tightness had returned. I felt frustrated by this unusual retightening and began to explore other areas that might be triggering this response.

When I looked at her left cheek, just in front of her ear, I noticed that the skin was flat, whiter than the rest of her face, with the diameter of a quarter. I asked if she knew what that whitish area was. She said that when she was three, she had fallen against a hot cookstove, and the whitish area was what remained of the burn scar.

I gently touched and palpated the scar tissue. At first, there was no sensation. But in a moment or two, she began to experience intense, excruciating pain. At the same time, she began to feel strong sensations radiating down into her neck and left arm.

Gradually the pain in the scar tissue and the sensations down her neck eased. As I worked on the scar tissue, it came into her mind that her left neck and arm had "always been weak" since childhood.

At the next session, she reported that there had been only a slight return of tightness in her neck and back. After a few more sessions, she was discharged, pain and symptom free.

I was astonished that a scar that had occurred fifty years earlier could hold so much pain and cause significant physical dysfunction. It certainly demonstrated the importance of examining and treating scar tissue.

Case History 2

A woman called and said it was becoming increasingly difficult for her to swallow. Food and medicine stuck in her throat. The problem had become increasingly severe over the past several months. Doctors thought her problem was caused by panic attacks, but she felt she panicked when she couldn't swallow. She heard of my work and asked if I could help her. I told her to get a doctor's referral, and we set up an appointment.

I carefully checked the tissues of her throat and detected a small, hard area on the left side. It felt like a scar. I asked her about it, and she said that several years earlier her neck had been cut by some falling glass. When I pressed on the scar, she felt sensations radiating into her throat. The scar responded rapidly to care and in two weeks had completely softened. By the end of this treatment period, she could swallow normally without any difficulty.

Case History 3

I was treating a woman for an upper extremity problem. During one session, I discovered a bit of hard tissue about the diameter of a quarter at the front of her chest just below her collarbone.

As I gently palpated this area, she began to cough violently. She told me she was a real estate agent and was frequently embarrassed when she was with clients by paroxysms of severe coughing that lasted for several minutes. This had been going on for years, but she had not been aware of this cough-triggering bit of tissue.

In the process of treatment I found that if I pressed on it, she began to cough. For the next several sessions, I worked to normalize this scarlike tissue. As it gradually softened, the violence of her reactive coughing lessened. Finally, the coughing completely ceased. At the

I carefully checked the tissues of her throat and detected a small, hard area on the left side. It felt like a scar. The scar responded rapidly to care and in two weeks had completely softened. By the end of this treatment period, she could swallow normally without any difficulty.

last session, the cause of her problem suddenly came into her mind. She recalled that when she was three she had had a severe case of whooping cough. She remembered the bouts of violent coughing and how it made her chest hurt.

Apparently, the trauma of coughing had injured her tissues and caused a scar to form. The scar had then retriggered the coughing episodes when the stress of dealing with clients caused the tissues surrounding the scar to tighten.

She called a few months later to let me know that she no longer experienced the embarrassing coughing episodes.

These three cases demonstrate the importance of reducing all scar tissue early on so future complications can be avoided.

The Schatz Technique™ Instructions

Scar tissue can trigger pain and physical dysfunction. All scar tissue, whether caused by burns, trauma, or surgical incisions, should be treated and released, thereby avoiding this possibility. *The Schatz Technique™* applied movements such as rippling, circles, back-and-forths, kneading, and nudges are effective; refer to the glossary for instructions.

Start your treatment sessions with extreme gentleness, as there may be considerable hidden pain locked up in the scar. Work slowly, be patient, and allow plenty of time. If the scar is thick and extensive, be prepared to treat in extended sessions for several weeks or months.

Sciatica

(And the Case of the "Torn Tensor Fascia Lata")

When the tissues of the gluteal area become tight and contracted, the pain receptors there are squeezed, causing the sensation of pain. The sciatic nerve passes through the region; therefore, doctors call pain in that area sciatica. However, tissue dysfunction rarely occurs in just one small area of the body.

Case History

A man in his late thirties was referred for treatment of severe sciatica. When I chatted with him before treatment, I learned that his painful sciatica had been developing over the past several months but that he had another problem that had been plaguing him for four years.

He told me he formerly enjoyed participating in martial arts but four years earlier had torn his tensor fascia lata when doing a karate kick. This injury forced him to stop his martial arts activity.

The tensor fascia lata is a thick, tough band of connective tissue that runs from the hip down to the knee. It is frequently involved in hip and knee problems but is so tough I could not imagine a karate kick could "tear it." I asked him how he knew it was torn. He said that, at the time, he was living in Boston and, as he wanted to have the very best care for his athletic injury, he went to the physician treating a particular athletic organization of great basketball renown. The doctor diagnosed his problem as a "torn tensor fascia lata."

The doctor prescribed a course of treatment consisting of ultrasound, heat, massage, exercise, and stretching. This regimen was diligently pursued for six months, but the pain and other symptoms worsened to such an extent that treatment was eventually discontinued. Nothing else was offered, so my patient continued to live in severe pain during the intervening years.

When I examined him, I found that the tissues of his gluteal area, particularly on the right side, down his right thigh and into his right knee, were contracted and painful to light touch. The tissues adjacent to his tensor fascia lata were particularly painful.

I asked him if his current doctor thought there might be some relationship between his "torn" tensor fascia lata and his painful sciatica. He told me he had wondered that himself, but his doctor said no, they were two distinctly separate issues.

I treated him intensively three times a week for two weeks. At the end of that time, he no longer had sciatic pain, and the symptoms relating to his tensor fascia lata had diminished.

He told me he was interested in getting every iota of his tensor fascia lata problem eliminated until there was not the slightest "twinge" of a problem. So we continued treatment, at decreasing frequency, for a total of three months. At the end of this time, he did not have the slightest twinge, and I discharged him from treatment, completely pain-and symptom-free, pleased and happy.

I called him two years following discharge, and he reported that there had been no return of either sciatica or tensor fascia lata pain. He had not returned to martial arts but felt he was physically able to do so now.

Here is an example of a doctor in charge of athletes, displaying the same ignorance of soft tissue dysfunction that doctors in charge of the general population display. If my patient had been a professional athlete, dancer, or other specialized performer, his career would have been ruined. Think of all the unfortunate individuals whose careers have been ruined.

The Schatz Technique™ **Instructions**

Refer to "Back Pain" for appropriate treatment techniques. For treatment of the tensor fascia lata, refer to "Knee Pain."

Shin Splints

The job assigned to the muscle group located at the shin is to lift the foot at each step. Unfortunately, this muscle, the tibialis anterior, is a small one and is easily overworked by the strenuous process of running. Over time, this muscle and its associated tissues becomes contracted, thickened, and painful. Doctors refer to this condition as shin splints. However, as with most soft tissue problems, other tissue areas become involved. Indeed, by the time an individual experiences pain and dysfunction of the shin tissues, the entire lower extremity has become dysfunctional.

Doctors, however, attempt to treat shin splints with rest, drugs, and, believe it or not, surgery! Directing attention and treatment exclusively to the area of the shin is to render a gross disservice to the athlete. To mutilate those dysfunctioning tissues with a sharp scalpel demonstrates a high level of ignorance. Proper treatment is to soften and normalize all dysfunctioning tissue so pain will go away and the body can become healthy once again.

Case History

I received a call from someone who said he was a serious runner. He had been unable to run for the past two weeks because of severe shin splints. The problem had plagued him for some time but had worsened over the past three months. He had been to a few doctors, but they had been unable to help him.

198

His immediate concern was an upcoming ten-mile run only one week away. He had his heart set on participating in the event, but, because of his painful shins, he feared he would not be able to run. Someone had mentioned my work, and he was calling to ask if I could help. I told him to get a doctor's referral that would enable me to examine and treat. We then set up an appointment for the following day.

When I examined him, I found that all the tissues of both his lower extremities were tight and contracted, particularly so from his knees down through his ankles and into his feet. The tissues of both calves were extremely tight and painful to mild examination. But most dysfunctioning of all was the condition of the tissues of his shins, which were almost as hard as wood. The skin was tightly adherent to underlying tissues. When I applied lotion, I could feel thick, well-defined, fibrotic bands throughout. The lightest examination caused excruciating pain.

I felt I could help him with a series of treatments, but was uncertain if we should start so soon before his important event. My treatment, by softening and normalizing his contracted tissues, could possibly bring to the surface considerable amounts of hidden pain that his body had accommodated itself to, which would make the ten-mile run, now only five days off, even more difficult to tolerate. On the other hand, the softened and normalized tissues might become completely pain-free and he could run without difficulty. It is difficult to predict the tissue response of the first few treatments.

After discussing the matter with me, he decided to go ahead with a treatment, because he certainly was unable to run in his present condition. The tissues of his thighs and calves softened considerably. The tissues of his shins, however, were more resistant, and did not soften to the same extent. At the end of the treatment, he said that his legs were free of pain and were "feeling pretty good." That was on Monday.

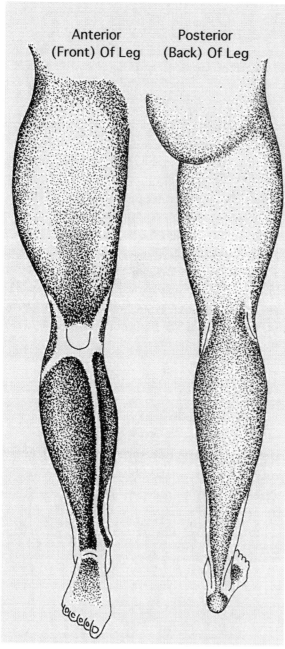

Anterior
(Front) Of Leg

Posterior
(Back) Of Leg

Extensive areas of tissue dysfunction
underlie what is called "shin splints."

He called the next Wednesday to give me a status report. His legs were completely pain-free the evening of the treatment, but on Tuesday morning he experienced moderate pain in both shins. This pain eased as the day went on. When he awoke on Wednesday morning, his legs were free of pain and he thought he would try a five-mile run. He finished his five miles without any pain or discomfort, but afterwards began to feel some pain creeping back.

Again, there was the dilemma of whether or not to give another treatment before the ten-mile run on Saturday. I felt that it might be best to hold off until after the run. He was feeling pretty good and I didn't want to take a chance of releasing more hidden pain.

He called on Monday to say that the ten-mile run went well, and that he had no pain or discomfort. I was greatly relieved to hear this. After this, I treated him for one month. The tissues of his shins and calves softened appreciably, and we extended treatment up to his hips. When discharged, he was running well with no complaints. I told him to call if he had any recurrence of symptoms. That was several months ago. No call yet.

The Schatz Technique™ Instructions

Soft tissue dysfunction that underlies the condition called shin splints can extend from the hips (or even higher) down into the ankle and foot. Those dysfunctioning tissues are also causative of knee pain. For *The Schatz Technique™* treatment suggestions, refer to "Knee Pain."

An important word of caution! Whenever treating your lea, particularly your calf, check first to see if it seems unusually warm, red or swollen. If so, do not treat and see your doctor immediately. This could be a sign of a serious health condition known as DVT (deep vein thrombosis) that could be life-threatening. Indeed, even if these warning signs are absent, 1 strongly suggest that readers visit their doctors before treating their legs to rule out any possibility of having this condition.

Sinus Pain

Several years ago, I was treating a young man for an upper extremity problem. One day, he came to my office complaining of excruciating sinus pain. The pain was so severe he was in tears. The only thing I could think to do was to have him lie down and to gently place my hands on his face where he was hurting. This seemed to give him some relief, so I was encouraged to move my fingers in small circles on both sides of his face adjacent to his nose, the areas of his pain. To my surprise and his delight, he reported that his pain was receding and he could feel that his sinuses were draining. Since that time, I have successfully treated a number of patients who have complained of sinus pain.

Case History

I was once the owner of a large rehabilitation group in Southern California and needed to hire a physical therapist for a particular treatment center. I knew of an excellent therapist and took him to lunch. When I discussed the position, he said he was fairly satisfied with his present job. Besides, he informed me that he was at the moment experiencing excruciating sinus pain and was finding it difficult to concentrate. He told me that he had suffered severe sinus pain for several years and nothing had helped the problem. I asked, if I were able to effectively treat his sinus pain, would he come to work for me? He answered with an emphatic "yes!"

We stopped by my office, and I proceeded to treat his sinuses (after he had called his doctor to get the permission necessary for me to treat him). As I did, I gathered from his demeanor that he was skeptical of what I was doing. At the end of forty minutes, he reported that there was no change in the amount of pain he was experiencing, and he left the office. I was extremely embarrassed by the lack of results.

However, later that afternoon he called and said that I had myself a therapist. Two hours after the treatment, he felt his sinuses open and drain. He said, "I don't know what you did, but it sure worked."

I gave him six more treatments. His sinus tissues were then soft, supple, and symptom-free. He readily learned to treat his own sinuses when retightening began, so there was no recurrence of pain or any other symptom in the three years he worked for me.

The Schatz Technique™
Instructions

The triangular shaped wedges of tissue that lie on either side of the nose are what I call the "sinus areas." (Also see page 203.) When lotion is applied to these areas, thick, fibrotic skin and underlying tissue is invariably revealed. When these thickened tissues are softened and normalized, symptoms of pain and congestion recede and disappear.

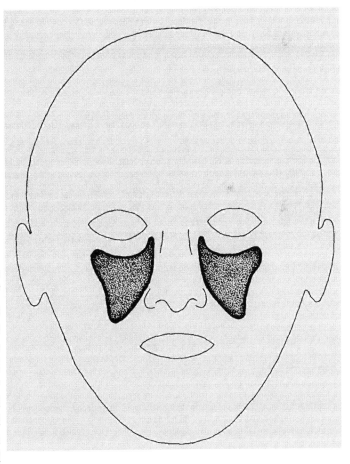

Dysfunctioning areas that cause sinus pain

203

The Schatz Technique™

Lie on your back with your upper body comfortably propped up by pillows or a bolster. Have lotion and a cup of warm water standing by. Apply a small amount of lotion to each wedge and explore. Begin your exploration using your forefingers as probes. Use circles, back-and-forths, and nudges as described in the glossary.

Is one side thicker? Is one or both hard and stiff? Do you find small, hard knots? These are bits of fibrotic tissue that will soften as treatment proceeds.

Place a finger next to your nose and run your thumb across the skin of a wedge. Is the skin thick? Does the skin ripple as your thumb is drawn toward your finger, or is it bound down to underlying tissue? Try the other wedge. Is the skin thicker? Less thick? More adherent to underlying tissues? Less adherent?

Grasp a wedge between thumb and forefinger. Can you move it about, or is it too thick and stiff? Can you nudge it with your forefinger? Try slow nudges, fast nudges. How about the other side, any difference?

If the lotion is drying out and getting sticky, add a bit more, or a drop or two of water, to get it slippery again. Perhaps you like the extra friction that you have with the drying lotion; it helps grip the skin when you maneuver it. If so, don't add lotion or water; use the friction to your advantage.

Explore each wedge thoroughly, from nose to cheekbone, and up and down-from the outer corner of your eye to the bottom of your cheekbone. Take your time; don't rush. When you have gained a sense of the tissues of your sinus areas, begin the treatment.

Reapply lotion, place your thumb under your jawbone for leverage, and sweep your finger slowly across the first wedge to be treated, down from the bone under your eye. Continue these sweeps until the entire wedge is covered. Take your time; don't rush. Repeat the movement several times. Keep your thumb where it is and use your finger to perform small circles over the wedge. Gradually enlarge the circles until each circle covers the entire wedge. Perform this movement several times. Is the wedge of tissue beginning to soften, to feel lighter? Now treat the wedge with small nudging movements.

Run your finger horizontally along the bone under your eye, from nose to cheekbone. Do you feel very small, hard, fibrotic knots in the skin and underlying tissues? These not only cause "bags" to form under your eyes but are also components of sinus problems. Treat these knots with small circles and up-and-downs. These tissue dysfunctions are stubborn and will require additional treatments before they soften and normalize. After gently treating one sinus wedge, move over and gently treat the other one.

Response to treatment varies widely. The effect can be immediate and dramatic, such as severe pain reduced to zero in a matter of minutes. At other times, a response is felt thirty minutes, or perhaps two or more hours, following treatment. I have had patients, treated in the morning, call late in the afternoon to tell me that their sinuses had just "opened" and were draining, with significant relief of pain. Some cases were more stubborn and required several visits. As with all soft tissue dysfunction, it is best to continue treatments until the tissues are soft and normalized, so symptoms are not likely to return.

Sinus Headache

Although many patients refer to their pain as "sinus headaches," their doctors deny the occurrence of sinus-generated headaches. In my experience, it is the patients who are correct. When a patient complains of sinus headache, I first check the "sinus areas" adjacent to both sides of the nose. I move out from these to investigate other areas for tight, fibrotic tissue. These are usually found on the face, frequently at the temporal and forehead areas, although the scalp, neck and upper back may also be involved. When all of these are reduced and normalized, the sinus headaches go away.

Case History

A woman in her late fifties came to me because of excruciating sinus pain she had endured for several years. She also suffered from what her doctors diagnosed as severe migraine headaches. The two problems were thought by her doctors to be separate. Over the years, she had been given various medicines and painkillers, all to no avail. The sinus pain and headaches grew worse and worse.

Finally, extensive surgery on her sinus cavities was performed. Sadly, this surgery also had no effect on her excruciating sinus pain and headaches, which continued unabated. Someone told her of my work, and she obtained the necessary doctor's referral.

When she reported for treatment, she stated that she was experiencing severe sinus pain and a severe headache. My examination revealed that the tissues overlying the left side of her face and cheek were hard, indurated, and extremely painful to the touch. I found contracted, fibrotic tissue extending from her sinus area to her left temple and up into her scalp. She reported that when I palpated these tissues her headache immediately worsened. She stated that none of the doctors, over the several years they had treated her, had ever examined or touched any of them. The triangular-shaped wedges of tissue that lie on either side of the nose are what I call the "sinus areas." (also see page 199) When lotion is applied to these areas, thick, fibrotic skin and underlying tissue is invariably revealed. I worked on the tight, contracted tissues, and as I did so, she reported that her sinus and headache pain was decreasing. By the end of the first treatment, she no longer had any pain whatsoever. She felt this was a miracle. I gave her two more treatments and discharged her, pain-free and very happy. I checked with her two years later, and she reported that she remained free of any pain.

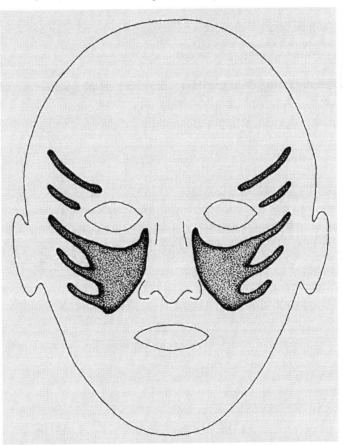

Dysfunctioning areas that cause sinus headache pain

The Schatz Technique™ Instructions

Lie on your back with your upper body comfortably propped up by pillows or a bolster. Have lotion and a cup of warm water standing by. Apply a small amount of lotion to each wedge and explore. Begin your exploration using your forefingers as probes. Use circles, back-and-forths, and nudges as described in the glossary.

Is one side thicker? Is one or both hard and stiff? Do you find small, hard knots? These are bits of fibrotic tissue that will soften as treatment proceeds.

Place a finger next to your nose and run your thumb across the skin of a wedge. Is the skin thick? Does the skin ripple as your thumb is drawn toward your finger, or is it bound down to underlying tissue? Try the other wedge. Is the skin thicker? Less thick? More adherent to underlying tissues? Less adherent?

Grasp a wedge between thumb and forefinger. Can you move it about, or is it too thick and stiff? Can you nudge it with your forefinger? Try slow nudges and fast nudges. How about the other side, any difference?

If the lotion is drying out and getting sticky, add a bit more, or a drop or two of water, to get it slippery again. Perhaps you like the extra friction that you have with the drying lotion; it helps grip the skin when you maneuver it. If so, don't add lotion or water; use the friction to your advantage.

Explore each wedge thoroughly, from nose to cheekbone, and up and down-from the outer corner of your eye to the bottom of your cheekbone. Take your time; don't rush. When you have gained a sense of the tissues of your sinus areas, begin the treatment.

Reapply lotion, place your thumb under your jawbone for leverage, and sweep your finger slowly across the first wedge to be treated, down from the bone under your eye. Continue these sweeps until the entire wedge is covered. Take your time; don't rush. Repeat the movement several times. Keep your thumb where it is and use your finger to perform small circles over the wedge. Gradually enlarge the circles until each circle covers the entire wedge. Perform this movement several times. Is the wedge of tissue beginning to soften and feel lighter? Now treat the wedge with small nudging movements.

Run your finger horizontally along the bone under your eye, from nose to cheekbone. Do you feel very small, hard, fibrotic knots in the skin and underlying tissues? These not only cause "bags" to form under your eyes but are also components of sinus problems. Treat these knots with small circles and up-and-downs. These tissue dysfunctions are stubborn and will require additional treatments before they soften and normalize.

After treating one sinus wedge, move over and treat the other one. After both wedges have been treated, finish with a gentle "towel rub."

After doing the techniques for normalization of the sinus areas, then explore and treat other areas of your face and head. You might also have to investigate your neck, upper back, and chest. If this is necessary, review *The Schatz Technique*™ treatment suggestions under "Migraine and Muscle Contraction Headaches."

Sprained Ankle

It is important to keep an open mind about any treatment model. Once practitioners get locked into a certain concept, they find it exceedingly difficult to let go of it. Take, for example, the treatment of sprained ankles.

Case History

At the end of her second week of treatment, a woman I was treating for an upper extremity problem came in one morning, limping painfully.

"Oh, no," I said. "What's happened now?"

She said her arm was fine but she had slipped the night before and sprained her ankle. She had just been to her doctor, who had examined her and wrapped her ankle in an Ace bandage. She hoped I could help and, knowing the system, had obtained a referral from her doctor.

I said there was nothing I could do for a sprained ankle. I then recited the conventional wisdom about the treatment of a sprained ankle: "cold, then heat, plenty of rest, elevation, gradual weight bearing as tolerated." She persisted, however, in her request that I do something, or, at least, try to do something for her ankle. Finally, I relented.

I unwrapped and examined her ankle. It was swollen and painful for her to move. However to my surprise, when I palpated the tissues well above the ankle on up into her calf and then down into her heel and instep, I found the tissues in these areas to be spasmed and painful to light touch. I thought, "Why not try to soften these spasmed and painful areas?" So I proceeded to gently work on them. They responded quickly and in a few minutes began to relax and soften.

After thirty minutes, I asked her to get up and see how her ankle felt. To her delight and to my surprise, she no longer had any pain or discomfort. She thanked me and walked out without a limp. Since then, I have treated four other patients with ankle sprains and got similar results.

What do these experiences point toward? Contrary to the commonly held assumption that it is the tendon at the ankle that is sprained when a "sprained ankle" occurs, I contend it is the soft tissues (muscles and fascia) attached to the tendon that are injured. When these fragile

Contrary to the commonly held assumption that it is the tendon at the ankle that is sprained when a sprained ankle occurs, I contend it is the soft tissues (muscle and fascia) attached to the tendon that are injured. When these fragile tissues are traumatized, they spasm.

tissues are traumatized, they spasm. The spasm squeezes nerves and vascular structures, which in turn produces the pain and swelling. Tendons are strong and tough, not easily injured or susceptible to being sprained, whereas soft tissues by their very nature are susceptible to injury.

The Schatz Technique™ Instructions

It never hurts to try, if you try in a gentle manner. My experience with treating sprained ankles has been limited but interesting. I see no harm in having others try similar gentle techniques. I urge you to have your injury checked to rule out the possibility of a fracture or some other severe injury before you start self-treatment.

Let's assume that your right ankle is affected. Lie on your left side with your upper body propped up on pillows or a bolster. This is so you can reach your ankle easily. Place some towels under the leg you are going to treat. Bend your knee and position your leg so it is as comfortable as possible. Apply some lotion to your calf up by your knee. Dilute it with a few drops of water so your treating hand can move gently and smoothly, without any friction, over the surface of your skin. Lubricate your entire leg from knee to toes in a similar manner.

Make gentle floats starting from about three inches above your ankle on up to your knee. Do this so gently that it causes no additional pain. If you feel increased pain, you probably are not doing it gently enough. Continue with these floats so all tissue surface is covered. Reposition your leg as necessary. If at any time you feel increased pain from what you are doing, back off and float with an even lighter touch. If even your lightest touch causes increased pain, then discontinue treatment. However, if you find that your tissues are relaxing and the pain is easing, then continue with the floats. With continued tissue relaxation, gently increase the intensity of treatment.

Now place your palm and fingers gently on your calf up by your knee, and, keeping them on that same spot, make gentle circles so that the deeper tissues there are gently moved. How did that feel? If it caused pain, then move even slower, with even more gentleness. If things are going well, move to another spot and do the same.

Continue until all tissues from knee to above the ankle have been moved in this gentle manner. If all is going well, then place your hands on opposite sides of the calf and make small circles in unison so that the tissues deep inside the calf are gently moved. Picture in your mind that you are gently moving your deeper calf tissues around your shinbone. Do you think your tissues are loosening? If so, increase the arc of the circles.

Now move down to the ankle itself. Gently place your palm on the outside of your anklebone. Don't do any moving; just place it there. How does it feel? If it doesn't hurt, make tiny, gentle circles with your palms. No pain? Then continue; if it hurts, discontinue. Now try the inside anklebone. If it feels okay, continue; if it hurts, discontinue.

212

Move down to your foot. Perform the same palmings. Continue until all areas of your foot have been gently treated. To finish, go back up to your knee and work down with circles. How do things feel now? They should feel better, and you should be more relaxed and feel less pain. Remember, at the slightest increase in pain, discontinue.

An important word of caution! Whenever treating your leg, particularly your calf, check first to see if it seems unusually warm, red or swollen. If so, do not treat and see your doctor immediately. This could be a sign of a serious health condition known as DVT (deep vein thrombosis) that could be life-threatening. Indeed, even if these warning signs are absent, I strongly suggest that readers visit their doctors before treating their legs to rule out any possibility of having this condition.

Tendinitis

Doctors blame tendons for all sorts of body pain. However, tendons are rarely a problem. The medical misdiagnosis of tendinitis is invariably bestowed upon individuals that suffer soft tissue dysfunction well away from the tendons and their protective sheaths. It springs from a lack of knowledge of soft tissue dysfunction. If doctors began carefully touching the bodies of their patients, they would understand this. Doctors attempt to treat misdiagnosed tendinitis with splints, medication and surgery.

Case History

The manager of a fast-food restaurant was referred for treatment. He brought in a referral bearing the diagnosis "tendinitis, both heels." The young man told me he experienced severe, excruciating pain with each step. He had a bandage wound around each ankle to limit motion there. His shoes were loosely laced because of dreadful pain in both feet, and he walked slowly as if in severe pain.

I examined his legs and feet and found that the tissues of both legs from calf down through forefoot and into his toes were tight, contracted, fibrotic, and severely painful to the lightest examination. Here was another case of extensive soft tissue dysfunction.

I told him I could feel contracted tissues and fibrotic fibers in his calves and feet and that there was a good possibility I might be able to help him by softening, releasing, and normalizing the dysfunctioning tissues. He said to go ahead with the treatment program I outlined.

I treated him for two weeks, three times a week. By this time, the affected tissues were normalized, and he was free of all pain. He walked quickly with no discomfort. When I discharged him at the end of the six sessions, he told me that at the first treatment, when I spoke of fibrotic fibers, he thought I was crazy because the whole thing sounded wacky. But now he had to admit that what I did had worked. Once again, tendons were blamed for what was really an extensive soft tissue problem.

The Schatz Technique™ Instructions

Doctors may mistakenly blame tendons for pain occurring anywhere in the body. Shoulders, elbows, hands, and heels are frequently misdiagnosed as having tendinitis. Refer to "Carpal Tunnel Syndrome" and "Shin Splints" for treatment suggestions. If you have been diagnosed as having tendinitis in another area of your body, refer to the appropriate section for treatment suggestions.

Tennis Elbow

Soft tissue dysfunction underlies complaints of body or headache pain and dysfunction, and usually the dysfunction is extensive in nature. This is true for what is commonly called "tennis elbow." Pain noted at the elbow is merely the tip of an extensive iceberg of soft tissue dysfunction. Tight and contracted tissues of the entire upper extremity and throughout large areas of the body are likely involved. When the dysfunctioning tissues are properly treated, the pain perceived at the elbow will go away.

Case History

A fifty-eight-year-old woman was referred for treatment. Her doctor had diagnosed her condition as tennis elbow. When I examined her, I found that the tissues of both upper extremities, neck, head, scalp, upper back, lower back, gluteal areas, and both lower extremities from her hips down to her toes were thick, tight, contracted, and severely painful. The tissues of her back were so thickened that I could not palpate her spinal column. Her shoulders were pulled painfully forward by contracted chest tissues.

She suffered from ear pain and tinnitus. Her body was so painful that she could do mild yard work for only fifteen minutes before dreadful pain shot up her legs into her back. She could sleep for only two to three hours at a time before the pain throughout her body awakened her. Her legs demonstrated significant development of peripheral vascular disease. She suffered from painfully severe bunions, and the tissues of both her hands were tight, thick, and painful. Yet, notwithstanding the fact that her entire body was severely painful, her doctor had diagnosed her problem simply as "tennis elbow."

I worked on her for eight months. When she was discharged, all her symptoms were significantly reduced. She could sleep for four to five hours and work in her garden for two to three hours before needing a rest. Her ear pain and tinnitus was reduced, as was much of the pain in the rest of her body, including her formerly painful elbow.

Eventually, however, she had surgery performed on her bunions. Her tissue dysfunction had progressed over the entirety of her life. When I saw her, it had become so severe that I could only more or less "patch things up," although she was pleased with the results of the treatments.

The Schatz Technique™ **Instructions**

The diagnosis of tennis elbow is a frivolous one, as demonstrated by the above case history. You will have to examine your body to find your dysfunctioning tissues. The tissues of your entire upper extremity are probably affected, so carefully check and treat from shoulder to fingers as described in "Carpal Tunnel Syndrome." The tissues of your neck and back are also likely areas. Refer to those sections for *The Schatz Technique*™ suggestions.

Tinnitus

Tinnitus can be caused by a multitude of underlying problems that respond to medical treatment. However, after all medically understood problems have been ruled out, a large number of patients continue to experience severe symptoms and are told that "nothing more can be done." The continued suffering of these individuals may be caused by soft tissue dysfunction.

When I treat someone for neck and back problems, I frequently find that they also complain of tinnitus (a sensation of "ringing" in the ears), a feeling of stuffiness in the ears, and ear pain. Usually, the tinnitus is more severe in one ear. Investigation invariably reveals thickened, fibrotic tissue adjacent to the ear at the area of the attachment of the sternocleidomastoid muscle, the long muscle that runs from the sternum (the breastbone) to just behind the ear. As a matter of fact, the substance of this muscle itself is frequently thick tough, and hardened, especially where it attaches close to the ear.

A component of the neck and back treatment is directed toward the sternocleidomastoid and the area of its attachment close to the ear. I found that as this tissue softens, patients state that ear symptoms, including tinnitus, diminish significantly. At times, they report that they no longer have any tinnitus, although this improvement to date has only been temporary. I have not had the opportunity to treat tinnitus for extended periods,

218

because when the neck and back problems are successfully reversed, the patient is discharged; the reduction of tinnitus is a secondary benefit of treatment. I do not know for certain that tinnitus can be completely eliminated over a longer course of treatment specifically directed toward it, but I am confident that this could happen.

Case History

I treated a patient who suffered for years with loud ringing and uncomfortable pressure in her right ear.

When I first started treating the severe pain and tightness of her upper back and neck, her symptoms of tinnitus and pressure were "unbearable" and "terribly disruptive," as she put it. As treatment continued, at first twice a week and then every two to three weeks, she no longer had any symptom of pressure, and described her symptom of tinnitus as "usually mild," with occasional episodes at moderate levels. At times, she was completely unaware of any ringing.

As the excruciating body pain she experienced at the start of her care diminished and she came in for treatment less frequently, we spent just a few minutes of her two-hour treatment on her "tinnitus area." The improvement of her tinnitus problem slowed, as had the urgency to treat the problem. She was discharged from treatment when her back and neck pain was completely resolved, although she still experienced the reduced level of tinnitus.

The Schatz Technique™ Instructions

The primary area of soft tissue dysfunction that underlies tinnitus is the same as for ear pain, namely, the sternocleidomastoid muscle (see page 126). The tissues of the scalp, face, and upper back may also be involved. The treatment techniques are the same as for ear pain. It is likely that the fibrotic development at the attachment of the sternocleidomastoid, just behind the ear, will be very thick, and will require extended treatment.

Lie on your back with your head comfortably supported by pillows. Arrange them so your head is tilted forward; this will produce some slack in your sternocleidomastoids (see page 52 for diagram). Let us assume that your left ear is the affected one. You will turn your head to the left; this will further relax the muscle where it attaches behind your left ear.

Slip your right hand under your head so the palm of your hand supports the weight of your head. This will free your fingers and thumb to explore and treat. Start your treatment at the area of attachment with your first and second fingers held closely together, i.e., doubled. This makes them into a very effective probing instrument. Use them to perform circles and back-and-forths. Take your time; don't rush. Treat the entire area that surrounds your ear, paying particular attention to the tissue behind and below.

Are you finding thick tissue that becomes painful with gentle treatment? Move up into the scalp region. Let your fingers follow any pain or contracted areas. As you move outward, add multiple finger movements.

Go back to the attachment and examine the sternocleidomastoid itself. Move down and pincer it gently between thumb and bent forefinger as you go. Roll it gently, feeling for contracted, fibrotic or painful areas. Try some gentle single-finger circles, back-and-forths, and single-finger stationary presses. Move down to where the muscle attaches to the chest wall and examine and treat. Use single-finger, double-finger, and multiple-finger circles.

Explore and treat the tissues of your face. Let your fingers look for tight, contracted areas and for areas that cause any increase of your ear symptoms. Refer to "Ear Pain" for detailed instruction. For treatment of the upper back, refer to "Migraine and Muscle Contraction/Tension Headaches."

TMJ

Tight, contracted tissues **outside** a joint can radiate pain perceived to be coming from inside the joint. Doctors do not understand this and are therefore confused about the etiology of the pain they misnamed temporomandibular joint (TMJ) pain. Doctors mistreat TMJ pain and dysfunction with drugs, surgery and crude and painful stretching.

As mentioned above, TMJ can be accompanied by severe pain, and excruciating headaches can be generated. However, it can also occur without the onset of pain. Neurologic tissue located close to the temporomandibular joint can be irritated and cause symptoms of nausea and dizziness. When patients complain of these symptoms, doctors, in their ignorance of tissue dysfunction, blithely tell these unfortunates that they have "emotional" problems, and they are hustled off to psychiatrists.

The jaw swings loosely from the skull, allowing wide opening and side-to-side movement, necessary for chewing food. The joint that allows this free movement is the temporomandibular joint; it's held in place by muscles attached to it, but these muscles and associated tissues may become tight, contracted, and fibrotic. They cannot open fully, and pain and other symptoms may be generated. Proper treatment is to normalize the tight, contracted tissues. When this is done, the mouth opens fully and symptoms go away.

Case History

When I first came to Virginia, I heard of a plastic surgeon who was interested in finding a physical therapist who had experience in working with TMJ patients. I immediately phoned and told him I had such experience and was interested in treating patients with TMJ. I briefly outlined my nonsurgical approach that led to successful treatment of many patients that suffered jaw pain. I told him I would be pleased to stop by his office and discuss my treatment in greater detail.

He said he would not have time for such a conversation but would have his secretary take my name and phone number and would call me if the need ever arose.

Three years later, I received a call from a dentist who wanted to refer a patient suffering from severe TMJ who had been unresponsive to prior care. I asked how he had heard of me, and he said the plastic surgeon I had spoken to three years earlier had given him my name and phone number.

I told the dentist I would be pleased to treat his patient and that I was currently working with a modality called "microcurrent." I had used this electronic device for several months, had good results with it for a variety of problems, and it seemed promising in treating TMJ.

I told him my plan was to try the microcurrent intensively for two weeks. If it was not effective with this patient, then I would use techniques that I had found to be effective in the past. He said the plan was sound and that the patient already had a referral allowing me to treat, and that I could start any time.

I immediately set up an appointment with the patient, an eighteen-year-old woman. I learned that she had been suffering a severely painful jaw for two years. She could open her mouth about one inch, barely enough to eat small bits of soft food slowly, and even minimal opening caused an increase in pain.

In addition, she suffered from a severe and continuous headache that had lasted two years. Her headache was rated as ten on a scale of one to ten, and had started at the same time as her TMJ symptoms. Both problems progressed rapidly shortly after a severe emotional experience.

The plastic surgeon had performed two surgeries on her temporomandibular joints. The first one was an exploratory arthroscopic surgery, which was unsuccessful in providing any improvement of her problem.

Since her jaw pain, limited motion, and her severe headache continued, a second surgery was performed. This was an extensive surgery in which a long incision started from one side of her jaw, extended continuously behind her hairline, and around to the other side of her jaw. Everything had been laid open with the doctor's sharp scalpel.

Unfortunately, this second surgery was as unsuccessful as the first. The young woman told me the second surgery cost six thousand dollars. Both of these surgeries had been performed *after* my phone conversation with the surgeon. Only recently had she been told there was a physical therapist available who might be able to help her with nonsurgical treatment.

I will admit that I was saddened, disappointed, and more than a bit angry to think that this woman had been subjected to painful and expensive surgeries and had been allowed to continue to suffer all that pain and physical dysfunction for such a long time when the surgeon had known three years earlier that nonintrusive and considerably less expensive treatment was available. It was an example of what I call surgical mutilation-that is to say, *inexcusable* surgical mutilation!

When I examined her, I found that the tissues of her scalp, face, jaw, neck, and upper back were severely tight, contracted, and excrutiatingly tender to the lightest touch. The surgical scar was easily palpated. Touching it caused additional discomfort. She was in continuous pain, and the slightest movement of her jaw caused the pain to intensify greatly. She told me she was at that moment experiencing her constant headache. She spoke slowly, as if she were in severe pain.

I started the two-week course of microcurrent treatment. Unfortunately, it did not produce the results I had hoped for. So at the end of the two-week trial, I phoned the referring dentist and told him that the microcurrent hadn't worked and I was ready to start treatment using my regular techniques.

To my surprise, he told me to stop treatment. He said he had other things in mind. I reminded him that the original plan was a two-week trial of microcurrent and that I was confident I could help this young woman. But he said no, stop treatment.

I was disappointed. My knowledge of the treatments in vogue regarding TMJ led me to believe that this young woman would not be helped and she would continue to suffer severe pain and dysfunction. Nevertheless, I had no choice but to stop treatment.

However, I was haunted by the thought that this young woman was continuing to suffer. Also, once I start treating someone, I become dedicated to achieve success. I felt frustrated and guilty in this case.

After two years had passed, I decided to call the father of this young woman, now twenty, to see how she was doing. Her father told me she was the same. Same headache, same jaw pain, same physical dysfunction. I asked what the dentist had tried after he took me off the case. I learned that the young woman had been sent to a "pain management center" for one visit. She had been given some "pain medication" that hadn't helped her.

I told her father that I had been troubled because I hadn't been allowed to continue to treat his daughter, and if she was interested, I would like to try again. I told him I would not charge for my services, that my only motivation was to help her. I told him I would need a referral to treat if she decided to try again. He said he would call her and pass on my message.

She called back a few minutes later and said she did indeed want to try again. She said she could get a doctor's referral, and we set up an appointment for the next day.

When she came in for her treatment, she told me I only had one week to treat her, as she was about to leave the area. When I examined her, I found she still had severely tight and contracted tissues around both sides of her jaw and on around the back of her neck and up into her scalp. All these tissues were extremely painful to light examination.

I treated her for three consecutive days in two-hour sessions, without any significant response. There was some softening of the contracted tissue and some minimal improvement in jaw opening but no letup in the headache or pain when she moved her jaw.

However, when she came in for her fourth treatment, she told me that she no longer had a headache. *It was completely gone.* A few hours after the last treatment, the tight areas I had been working on had finally relaxed. In addition, she was now able to open her jaw enough to eat regular food without pain, although she did not have a completely full jaw opening. I only had the opportunity of treating her one more time before she moved away.

224

I spoke to her by phone one year later. She said that the headache had never returned, her jaw had remained relaxed, and she was continuing to eat regular food without any pain or discomfort. I told her to call me if she had any return of prior symptoms.

The Schatz Technique™ Instructions

Soft tissue dysfunction is the primary cause of TMJ pain. The problem is with tight, contracted, fibrotic tissues outside the joint. The pain radiates and is perceived to be coming from within the joint. As with most symptoms of soft tissue dysfunction, TMJ pain is usually an expression of an extensive problem. Look for tight, contracted, and painful tissues in the scalp, face, neck, and upper back. All these areas have to be examined, treated, and normalized. Review the treatment of these areas as described in "Migraine and Muscle Contraction Headaches," "Sinus Headache," and "Sinus Pain."

We will now concentrate on jaw tissue proper, usually the most important contributor of pain and physical dysfunction. The primary muscle that is responsible for chewing action, the masseter, begins just above the joint. It starts as a narrow band and widens as it descends to its attachment on the jawbone. When the masseter contracts, it brings the jaw up so food can be chewed. It is a strong muscle and, when it spasms, it grips your jaw tightly.

A misguided form of treatment is to attempt to *force* the jaw open. Doctors prescribe devices that are designed to do just that. They will stimulate your masseter to become even more painful and dysfunctional; it is a form of torture rather than treatment. And if doctors suggest surgery, tell them to read this book.

The proper treatment for any soft tissue dysfunction is to soften and normalize the tissue. Soften and normalize the masseter, and it will release its grip on your jaw and your pain will go away.

Start by placing the knuckles of your fingers against your cheek, using your thumb as the probe and treating instrument. Brace the elbow of your treating hand against the wrist of your other hand, which, in turn, is resting against your abdomen. This will give you leverage and prevent fatigue. Begin without lotion. The dysfunction of the masseter is usually so severe that you won't need the lotion to reveal the fibrotic formations, and the friction will allow you to use the skin to assist your probing. You will see what I mean once you try it.

Try circles with the tip of your thumb and then with the pad of your thumb. Alternate this from time to time. Go slowly, as the tissues here need a lot of care. I feel confident that you will immediately find thick, contracted, and fibrotic tissue that contains large amounts of pain. Now apply lotion and continue your explorations.

Move your examining hand so the thumb is placed in a stationary position under your jaw. This allows your forefinger to be used in a free-floating manner to find the outline of the masseter. The muscle is triangular-shaped and attaches to about half of the jawbone. Use your forefinger in side-to-side movements until you get a good idea of the masseter's boundaries, then focus your attention specifically on the muscle. Treat it thoroughly. It will

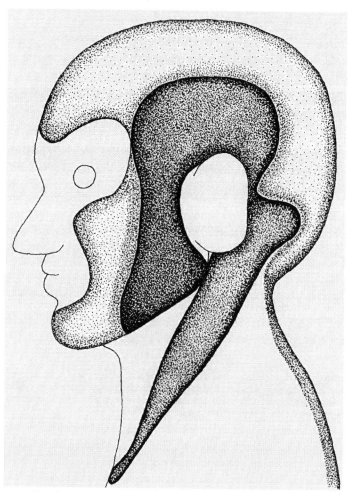

Dysfunctioning areas that cause TMJ problems

probably be painful to begin with, and will likely become even more tender once you start treating it, especially where it attaches up near the joint. Use single-, double-, and multiple-finger circles, back-and-forths, thumb and finger drags, ripples, and nudges.

Pay close attention to where the muscle attaches above the joint. Use firm double-finger probes, circles, and back-and-forths. Let your fingers follow wherever pain and tightness leads them, which is probably well up into your scalp.

Clench and release your teeth. This action will reveal all the areas of your scalp that are associated with your temporomandibular joint. You will be surprised how extensive this is. These tissues have to be examined, treated, and normalized. Use multiple-finger back-and-forths, circles, and nudges, and treat these areas thoroughly.

Now carefully examine and treat the masseter where it attaches to your jawbone. Double-finger back-and-forths along the length of your jaw will undoubtedly reveal well-defined fibrotic development in the form of hard wire like configurations running across the length of your jawbone. Follow them under the jaw line. Treat the tissues there by pincering with your thumb on the underside of your jawbone and the knuckle of your bent first finger on the other side. The first finger will remain stationary, and your thumb pad will perform circles and back-and-forths. These wire like formations will require several treatments to become fully normalized.

Turn your attention to the skin overlying your masseter. Use thumb sweeps and skin graspings. Look for thickened, adherent, and painful skin, particularly at the angle of your jaw. Use your thumb for skin rippling and nudgings there.

Response to treatment can vary. Two or three treatments may bring dramatic reduction in symptoms; however, several treatments are usually required to normalize the dysfunctioning tissues that are primarily responsible for the pain and difficulty in proper jaw movement. At times, response can be frustratingly slow, and several weeks or months (at reduced frequency of treatment) are needed to bring the desired results.

Trigger Finger

An individual may find that one of her fingers has developed a tendency to become locked into a bent position when she attempts to grasp an object. Doctors call this problem a "trigger finger." It is another example of the medical profession focusing on one small part of a patient's body to the exclusion of all the others. Doctors do not realize that all areas of their patient's body are marvelously interconnected.

The problem of trigger finger occurs when tissues of the palm become thick and fibrotic and press down tightly on finger flexors. When this happens, finger movement becomes erratic. However, these fibrotic areas are merely a small part of extensive tissue dysfunction. Doctors are unable to see the total picture. They are focused only on the fibrotic nodules; the rest of the body is unimportant and out of focus.

The problem of trigger finger occurs when tissues of the palm become thick and fibrotic and press down tightly on finger flexors. When this happens, finger movement becomes erratic. However, these fibrotic areas are merely a small part of extensive tissue dysfunction.

228

Case History

A professional artist living one hundred miles from my home heard about my work and called me. She told me she had a painful problem with her right hand, and that it was interfering with her work as an artist. She said her problem had been diagnosed as trigger finger and that it made it difficult for her to hold a brush and paint. She had been sent to a surgeon, a hand specialist, who first injected the area with cortisone, and when that was unsuccessful, had operated on it. Not only was the surgery unsuccessful but it also made the area more painful, and it was now more difficult to hold and manipulate a brush. She asked if I could help her. I told her that I would need a doctor's referral to check and treat her. She told me that would be no problem, and we made an appointment for later that week.

She arrived at the appointed time, bearing her referral. The surgeon who had performed the unsuccessful surgery on her hand had refused to write a referral allowing me to treat, but another doctor had signed one. When I examined her hand, I found that her fingers were swollen and were purplish in color. They moved slowly and stiffly. The skin of her palm was drawn tight. Her skin creases were deep and tender to examination.

I noted that the surgical scar in her palm was thick, adherent to adjacent tissue, and was painful to mild examination. I could feel the thickened tissue adherent to her finger flexors that was causing the trigger finger effect. I also found that the tissues extending from her hand up through her arm to her shoulder, neck, and back, were tight, contracted, fibrotic, and extremely painful to examination.

She responded well to treatment, and in ten sessions the tissues in her hand and fingers, and throughout her upper extremity, were soft, supple, and pain-free. She no longer had symptoms of trigger finger and could paint without any discomfort or disability. She was discharged, healthy and happy.

The Schatz Technique™ **Instructions**

For *The Schatz Technique*™ treatment suggestions, refer to "Carpal Tunnel Syndrome."

Whiplash and Other Accident Trauma

Soft tissues of the body immediately react to the trauma of a motor vehicle accident by going into spasm. Once spasm starts, it never releases, and becomes self-perpetuating. Spasmed tissue is the initiator of progressive pain and physical dysfunction, because unless properly treated, it gradually becomes contracted and then fibrotic.

In addition, as time passes, the local area that was originally injured, triggers other areas of the body to become affected. What was once a limited local problem becomes extensive and global. Unless properly treated, the pain and physical dysfunction that follow a motor vehicle accident can become what doctors call chronic.

If spasmed tissue is properly treated and released early on, the later stage of contraction and fibrosis can be avoided. The earlier effective treatment is initiated, the easier the problem is to treat, and the greater the assurance for a successful outcome.

However, even the late stage of development, the so-called chronic stage, responds to proper treatment. That is to say, even when body tissues have been allowed to become severely contracted and fibrotic, expectation of significant reversal of tissue dysfunction and its secondary symptom of pain is still high, although these cases are more challenging to treat.

230

I have frequently heard the comment, "Once you've been in a car accident, you're never the same again." Unfortunately, this is usually true, but if proper treatment is given, it doesn't have to be.

I will describe two cases, one in which timely treatment was given, and the other in which it wasn't, to make this point clearer.

Case History 1

A young woman was referred for treatment four days after her car was rear-ended. She presented with severe pain and tightness throughout her neck, back, chest, and both arms. She experienced severe and constant headaches. She was anxious and tearful and found it difficult to concentrate. Going into work was agonizing because of the severe pain, which worsened as the day went on.

When I examined her, I found that the tissues of her scalp, neck, back, upper chest, and both arms were severely spasmed and painful to even very mild examination. She said she was experiencing a very severe headache. She talked and moved slowly, as if she were in severe pain.

I treated her gently for two hours. I could feel the spasm reducing as I worked. At the end of the two-hour treatment, her headache was almost gone, her body pain was "a lot less," and she felt "much, much, better."

I continued to treat her, at decreasing frequency, for five weeks. At the end of this time, she was symptom-free, she had no chronic pain, and her tissues were soft and supple. She was discharged, happy and delighted.

Case History 2

A woman was referred to me two years after she had been injured in a motor vehicle accident. She also had been involved in a rear-end collision. She told me she had been treated with pain and anti-inflammatory medication. Her doctor had also prescribed a course of physical therapy consisting of hot packs, five minutes of massage, four or five minutes of ultrasound, and exercises and stretches. Her condition worsened as these treatments continued. By the end of each physical therapy session, her pain became "almost unbearable."

After four months of these treatments, her pain had developed into a constant agony. She couldn't bear another physical therapy session, and so she stopped going. She was criticized by her doctor and physical therapist for being "noncompliant," and this observation was duly noted in her medical record.

Since that time, she required as much pain medication as her doctor would allow, just to "barely survive." She was depressed, in constant pain, had frequent, severe headaches, and was at risk of losing her job because of frequent work absences. She was very concerned because her pain, unbearable as it was, was gradually getting worse and her body was getting ever tighter.

When I examined her, I found that the tissues of her scalp, neck, back, chest, and both arms were tight, thick, contracted and fibrotic. The skin overlying these areas was thickened, adherent to underlying tissues and was exquisitely tender to even the lightest touch.

Immediately following a very mild first treatment, her body reacted with a flare-up of excruciating pain throughout the treated area. It was one hour before things calmed down enough for her to leave my office. I apologized for the increased pain the treatment had caused, but she told me she was encouraged because her body felt a little "looser," and she could move a "little easier."

Following the first few treatments, she experienced increased pain, but at the same time, she noticed that her tissues felt looser and lighter. As treatments continued, she no longer experience increased pain; instead, her chronic pain lessened during and after each treatment.

I treated her in two-hour sessions, three times a week for the next three months. Gradually, her tissues became less thick, fibrotic, and painful. She was no longer missing work, and her quality of life had improved dramatically. I wanted to continue treating her, to normalize the significant areas of tissue dysfunction that remained, but she had to move away from the area.

I called her a year after treatments stopped. She told me she was doing "so-so." She could feel her body gradually retightening and had tried to find somebody in her area that treated the same way I did, but had been unsuccessful.

It is unfortunate this woman's body had been allowed to become severely contracted and fibrotic. If proper and effective treatment had been started early, it is likely that her pain and suffering could have been avoided.

The Schatz Technique™ **Instructions**

The primary areas to be treated for whiplash are the head, neck, upper back, and chest. Review "Migraine and Muscle Contraction Headaches" for instructions. If other areas of your body have been injured in a car accident, refer to the corresponding treatment sections.

Prevention:

The Healthcare of the Future Will Be

A World Without Chronic Pain

As the information in this book demonstrates, soft tissue dysfunction is the primary cause of chronic pain, from migraines to painful bunions. Physical and emotional insults stimulate the body to form contracted tissues that squeeze pain receptors and damage joint structures. The *process* starts in early childhood and progresses throughout the life of the individual.

The cause of chronic pain can be treated and normalized so pain and its accompanying physical disorder will go away and stay away. The sooner treatment is initiated, the more likely a complete reversal will occur. Sadly, the system of care presently in place does not provide treatment for any stage of this process.

A new healthcare system is needed, one that recognizes and treats tissue dysfunction, instead of dispensing dangerous drugs and performing drastic surgeries directed toward its secondary symptoms.

In the future, pain sufferers will not have to treat themselves. I envision a system that provides periodic "tissue checks." Practitioners will gently examine the body from head to toe. They will look for, identify, and treat *early* stages of spasm, before the health of the individual is compromised, *before* chronic pain occurs.

234

This will make for a healthier and happier population. There will be enormous savings because costly drugs, surgeries and the currently unproductive and repetitive provider visits will be eliminated. Individuals will be treated by practitioners who charge reasonable fees for good, honest work, instead of paying exorbitant fees to pseudo experts and high-priced surgeons.

In the future, pain sufferers will not have to treat themselves. I envision a system that provides periodic "tissue checks." Practitioners will gently examine the body from head to toe. They will look for, identify, and treat early stages of spasm, before the health of the individual is compromised, before chronic pain occurs.

For example, an article titled "What Is Carpal Tunnel Syndrome?" that appeared in the July 14, 1999, issue of *The Journal of the American Medical Association (vol.282, no. 2) states, "More than 200,000 carpal tunnel release surgical procedures are performed each year in the United States, which makes it the most common surgical procedure performed on the hand."*

The article points out that these procedures, estimated to cost more than one billion dollars per year, are performed without a clear diagnostic basis.

This means that in the next five years doctors will cut into one million carpal tunnels, at a cost to society of five billion dollars, yet all without diagnostic justification!

The practitioners of the healthcare of the future will look back at this period as the dark ages of chronic pain treatment. By keeping tissues healthy, symptoms of carpal tunnel syndrome that now occur in epidemic proportions will be a thing of the past. Billions of dollars will be saved by changing our treatment approach for this one condition alone.

Think of the many thousands of surgeries performed every year on necks, backs, hips, and knees that are directed toward the secondary symptom of pain not toward the problem that *caused* the pain and continues to undermine the health of the pain sufferer after the inappropriate surgery has been performed. Here, we get into astronomical amount of savings because inevitably the global aspects of tight, contracted body tissues profoundly degrade the earning potential of the pain sufferer, and the resulting cost to society from currently ineffective treatment is incalculable.

It is my contention that the majority of people who end up in nursing homes, wracked with pain and unable to care for themselves, are there because their bodies became progressively dysfunctional over a period of years—the end result of the present misguided and inappropriate healthcare system.

The practitioners of the future will understand the relationship between soft tissue dysfunction and organ systems that results in a lowered level of health. I have caught glimpses of this relationship. For example, I have observed central blood pressures drop significantly, for extended periods, by normalizing contracted tissues of the low back and gluteal region. This demonstrates a relationship between soft tissue dysfunction and the cardiovascular system. And if there is a relationship with the cardiovascular system, why not, then, with other systems of the body?

I believe the importance of treating soft tissue dysfunction early in life, before extensive damage takes place, before organ systems are affected, so bodies can remain healthy and free of pain will be appreciated and the present methods of mistreating soft tissue dysfunction with drugs and mutilating surgery will be discredited and discontinued. *I hope this book points the way to that healthcare of the future when chronic pain will be distant memory!*

About the Author

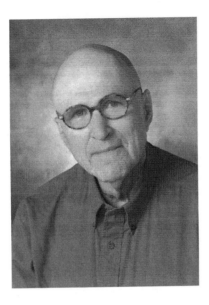

Bernard Schatz, P.T., has studied and treated chronic pain for over half a century–since 1950, when he began work at the Institute for Medical Research, Cedars of Lebanon Hospital, Los Angeles.

He discovered that the primary cause of chronic pain is contracted tissues that press on nerves. If contracted tissues occur in the neck and scalp, doctors call the pain a "migraine." If contracted tissues occur in the hand and arm, doctors call it "carpal tunnel syndrome," and if it occurs throughout the body, "fibromyalgia." It's one condition with many names.

Bernard developed a method, the Schatz Technique™ that normalizes contracted tissues. They become healthy and free of pain.

By the way, Bernard is 78 and has no pain anywhere in his body. In the past he suffered pain in his neck, shoulders, arms, back and legs. Pain that doctors called "chronic." However, he treated himself in the way he advises others. The result: for many years he wakes in the morning without pain, and goes through the day without pain. He walks with a spring in his step instead of hobbling around." (If he could do it so can readers of this book.)

Since this book was first published I have received emails and letters from people all over the world telling me how much my book has helped them. I want to thank them and hope that more and more people learn to help themselves and others. This information in the book provides the ground work to perform a basic touch. Some call it the "Schatz touch." The more one uses the information the more skilled and effective the touch becomes.

One person has followed through to learn all the complexities that my years of experience have developed. That person is JoAnn M. Christy. JoAnn, a massage therapist, started as an apprentice, and then joined me in my practice for two years.

At the age of seventy-eight, I am still practicing the technique that I love so much. It pleases me to know that there is someone else (more than thirty years younger) who has learned all there is to know about what I have discovered. JoAnn is indeed, a "Certified *Schatz Technique ™* Practitioner."

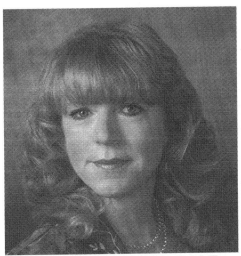

JoAnn M. Christy R.R.T., C.M.T.

JoAnn's email address is: Massage2Go@aol.com

By the way, if you hear of anyone besides JoAnn, who professes to perform "*The Schatz Technique™*" or presumes to be a " *Schatz Technique™* practitioner" you are now informed that they have not been authorized by me to do so.

Index

To purchase additional copies of this book for friends and family that suffer chronic pain or your health care professional, visit:

ReverseYourPain.com

Also visit the web site for more information on chronic pain.

Made in the USA
Lexington, KY
26 March 2010